TUNG ACUPUNCTURE POINTS

REFERENCE GUIDE

Also by Deborah Bleecker:

Insomnia Relief
Natural Back Pain Solutions
Acupuncture Points Handbook
Shingles Relief

TUNG ACUPUNCTURE POINTS

REFERENCE GUIDE

DEBORAH BLEECKER, LAC, MSOM

1st Edition
Draycott Publishing, LLC

ISBN-13: 978-1-940146-82-9

CONTENTS

Unnumbered Tung Points

Points in Pin Yin Order

Pin Yin	Number
Bei Mian	44.07
Bi Yi	1010.22
Bo Qiu	77.04
Ce San Li	77.22
Ce Xia San Li	77.23
Chang Men	33.10
Chong Xian	22.02
Chong Zi	22.01
Da Bai	22.04
Da Jian	11.01
Dan	11.13
Di Huang	77.19
Di Shi	33.14
Di Zong	44.09
Er Bei	99.07
Er Huan	99.01
Er Jiao Ming	11.12
Er San	99.08
Er Zhong	77.06
Fei Xin	11.11
Fen Jin	44.01
Fu Chang	77.12
Fu Ding	44.04
Fu Jian	11.03

Fu Ke	11.24
Fu Kuai	1010.15
Fu Yuan	11.22
Gan Mao Er	88.08
Gan Mao Yi	88.07
Gan Men	33.11
Guang Ming	77.28
Hai Bao	66.01
Hou Hui	1010.06
Hou Zhi	44.05
Hou Zhui	44.02
Hua Gu Er	55.03
Hua Gu San	55.04
Hua Gu Si	55.05
Hua Gu Yi	55.02
Huan Chao	11.06
Huo Bao	55.01
Huo Chuan	33.04
Huo Er	99.03
Huo Fu Hai	33.07
Huo Ju	66.11
Huo Lian	66.10
Huo Ling	33.05
Huo Quan	88.16
Huo San	66.12
Huo Shan	33.06
Huo Xi	11.16
Huo Ying	66.03

Huo Zhi	88.15
Huo Zhu	66.04
Jian Zhong	44.06
Jie Mei Er	88.05
Jie Mei San	88.06
Jie Mei Yi	88.04
Jie Xue	88.28
Jin Er	99.05
Jin Qian Shang	88.24
Jin Qian Xia	88.23
Li Bai	44.12
Ling Gu	22.05
Liu Kuai	1010.16
Liu Wan	66.08
Luo Tong	44.14
Ma Jin Shui	1010.13
Ma Kuai Shui	1010.14
Men Jin	66.05
Ming Huang	88.12
Mu	11.17
Mu Dou	66.07
Mu Er	99.02
Mu Fu	66.02
Mu Huo	11.10
Mu Liu	66.06
Mu Yan	11.20
Mu Zhi	1010.18
Nei Tong Guan	88.29

Nei Tong Shan	88.30
Nei Tong Tian	88.31
Pi Zhong	11.18
Qi Hu	77.26
Qi Huang	88.14
Qi Jiao	33.02
Qi Kuai	1010.17
Qi Men	33.01
Qi Zheng	33.03
Qian Hui	1010.05
Qu Ling	33.16
Ren Huang	77.21
Ren Shi	33.13
Ren Zong	44.08
San Yan	11.21
San Zhong	77.07
Shang Bai	22.03
Shang Chun	77.15
Shang Jiu Li	88.26
Shang Li	1010.09
Shang Liu	55.06
Shang Quan	88.22
Shang Zu	44.16
Shen Guan = Tian Huang Fu	77.18
Sheng Hui	1010.01
Shi Yin	88.32
Shou Jie	22.10

Shou Qian Jin	33.09
Shou Wu Jin	33.08
Shou Ying	44.03
Shui Er	99.06
Shui Jin	1010.20
Shui Jing	66.13
Shui Qu	66.09
Shui Shang	66.14
Shui Tong	1010.19
Shui Xian	66.15
Shui Yu	44.17
Si Fu Er	1010.10
Si Fu Yi	1010.11
Si Hua Fu	77.10
Si Hua Li	77.13
Si Hua Shang	77.08
Si Hua Wai	77.14
Si Hua Xia	77.11
Si Hua Zhong	77.09
Si Ma Shang	88.18
Si Ma Xia	88.19
Si Ma Zhong	88.17
Si Zhi	77.20
Tian Huang	77.17
Tian Huang	88.13
Tian Shi	33.15
Tian Zong	44.10
Tong Bei	88.11

Tong Guan	88.01
Tong Shan	88.02
Tong Shen	88.09
Tong Tian	88.03
Tong Wei	88.10
Tu Er	99.04
Tu Shui	22.11
Wai Jian	11.04
Wai San Guan	77.27
Wan Shun Er	22.09
Wan Shun Yi	22.08
Wu Hu	11.27
Xia Bai	22.07
Xia Chun	77.16
Xia Jiu Li	88.27
Xia Qu	44.15
Xia Quan	88.20
Xiao Jian	11.02
Xin Chang	11.19
Xin Men	33.12
Xin Xi	11.09
Yan Huang	11.23
Yi Zhong	77.05
Yu Huo	1010.21
Yun Bai	44.11
Zhen Jing	1010.08
Zheng Ben	1010.12
Zheng Jin	77.01

Zheng Shi	77.03
Zheng Zong	77.02
Zhi San Zhong	11.14
Zhi Shen	11.15
Zhi Si Ma	11.07
Zhi Tong	44.13
Zhi Wu	11.26
Zhi Wu Jin	11.08
Zhi Yan	11.25
Zhong Bai	22.06
Zhong Jian	11.05
Zhong Jiu Li	88.25
Zhong Quan	88.21
Zhou Huo	1010.23
Zhou Jin	1010.24
Zhou Kun	1010.03
Zhou Lun	1010.04
Zhou Shui	1010.25
Zhou Yuan	1010.02
Zong Shu	1010.07
Zu Qian Jin	77.24
Zu Wu Jin	77.25

INTRODUCTION

This book is a combination of the points and indications from multiple point books and online references. It includes over 110 points not included in the *Top Tung Acupuncture Points* book by Brad Whisnant. It does not include the clinical application notes by Brad, so please refer to that book for in depth notes. There are 163 point images in this book, many of which have not been published previously.

My goal with this book was to combine and cross reference books, and make an easy to use, practical guide. The book is sorted by point number, and it is easy to locate the points quickly. The first point location book I wrote is called *Acupuncture Points Handbook*, which is a cross-reference of numerous TCM books. I found a lot of discrepancies across different sources, as you will find with all acupuncture information. I have done my best to use the most common information. I cross-referenced location descriptions and included information that made the points easier to locate.

Included in this book is an index of the indications at the back. There is also a chart of the points sorted by Pin Yin name. Some teachers prefer to use the Chinese name for the points, so this chart makes it easy to find the point numbers quickly.

This book is meant to be a practical reference, as a helpful addition to other Tung books. It is meant to be a quick reference guide to the majority of the points. If you are new to Tung acupuncture, please refer to the references at the back of the book.

Treat Most Points on the Opposite Side

Most points are treated on the opposite side of the pain. If you are in doubt, treat the opposite side. Some points do not have an insertion depth listed.

Having the Patients Move during Treatment

When treating pain, many practitioners have the patient move after the needles are inserted.

11.01, 11.02, 11.03, 11.04

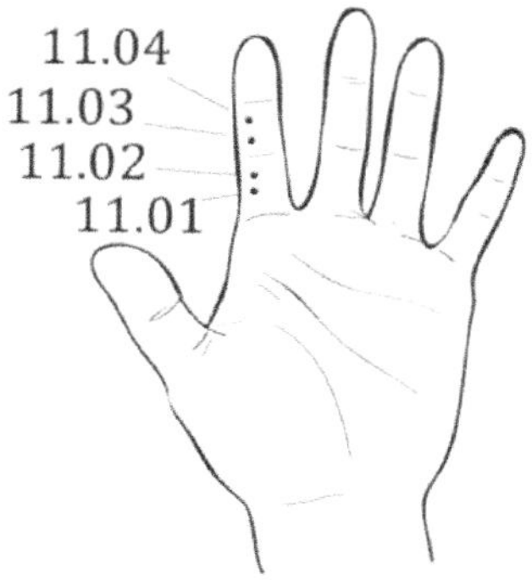

11.01, Da Jian, Big Distance

Indications: Heart disease, knee pain, hernia, pain in the inner canthus of the eye.

Location: On the index finger, .3 cun from the center of the finger, on the proximal section of the finger.

11.02, Xiao Jian, Small Distance

Indications: Bronchitis with yellow mucus, knee pain, chest stuffiness, palpitations, hernia, pain in the inner canthus of the eye, small intestine inflammation.

Location: On the index finger, .3 cun from the center of the finger, .2 cun distal to 11.01.

11.01, 11.02, 11.03, 11.04

11.03, Fu Jian, Floating Distance
Indications: Hernia, toothache, stomach pain, inflamed urethra.
Location: On the index finger. One fifth of a cun from the midline of the middle section of the finger. Insertion is .2 to .25 cun.

11.04, Wai Jian, Outer Distance
Indications: Hernia, toothache, inflamed urethra, and stomach pain.
Location: On the index finger, one fifth of a cun from the midline of the middle section of the finger, .66 cun from the distal crease. Insertion is .2 to .25 cun.

11.05

Zhong Jian - Center Distance

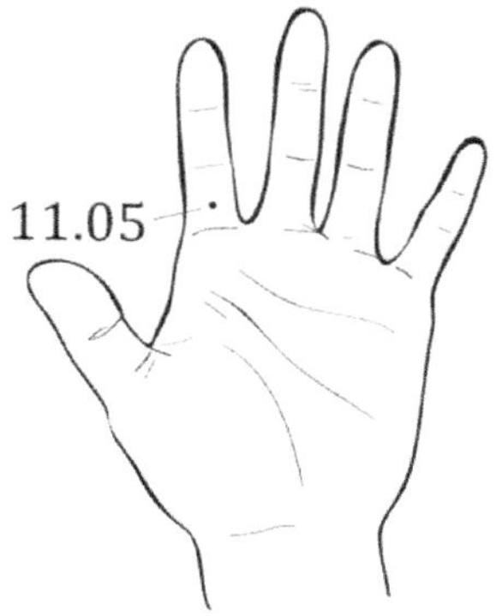

Location: In the center of the proximal section on the palmar side of the index finger.

Indications: Chest oppression, palpitations, knee pain, dizziness, and vertigo.

11.06

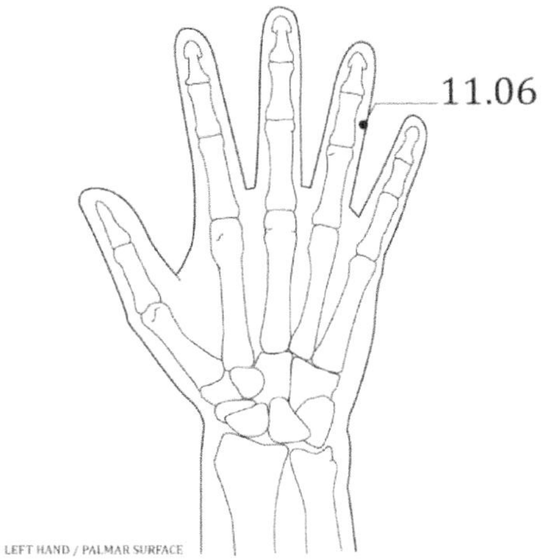

Huan Chao - Return To The Nest

Indications: Uterine pain, uterine tumor, and uterine inflammation, and irregular menstruation, leucorrhea with reddish discharge, fallopian tube obstruction, uterus retroversion, frequent urination, vaginal swelling, and frequent miscarriage, calms the fetus.

Reaction areas: Liver, Kidney

Location: On the palmar, and ulnar side of the middle segment of the ring finger, in the center between the 2nd and 3rd finger creases. Perpendicular insertion where the white and pink skin meet.

11.07

Huan Chao - Finger Rapid Horses

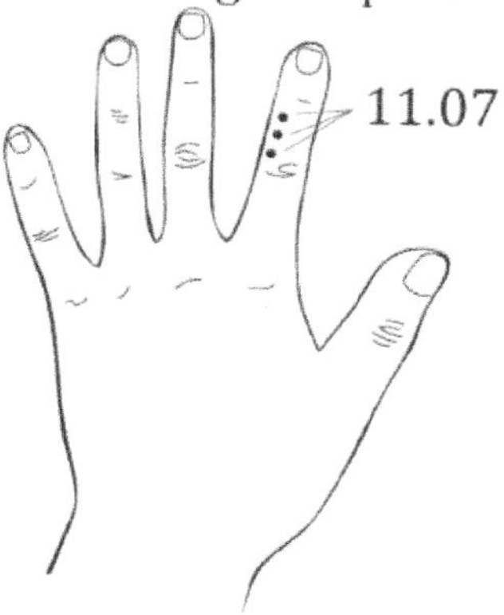

Indications: Pleurisy, pain of the pleura, dermatosis, dark spots on the face, rhinitis, tinnitus, and ear infection.

Location: Locate the first point .2 cun on the ulnar side the midline of the middle section of the dorsal side of the index finger. The second point is 0.3 cun above the first one and the third is 0.3 cun below it.

11.08

Zhi Wu Jin - Finger Five Metal

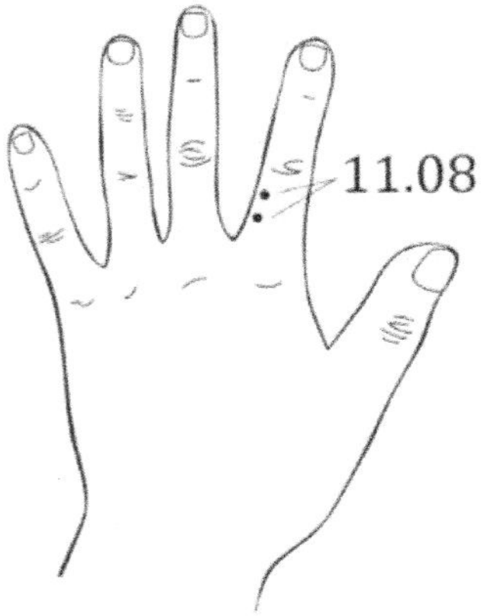

Indications: Intestinal inflammation, abdominal pain, and fish bone stuck in the throat.

Location: On the dorsum of the index finger, one fifth of a cun on the ulnar side of the midline of the proximal section.

11.09

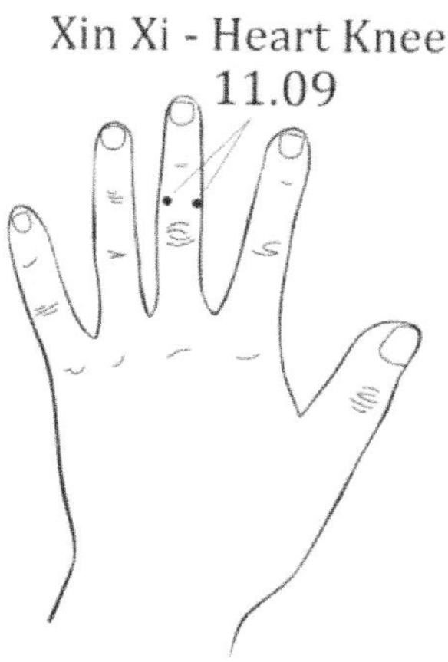

Indications: Knee pain and scapula pain, upper back pain, and shoulder pain.

Reaction area: Heart

Location: Located on both sides of the middle segment of the middle finger on the dorsal side, in the center between the second and third finger creases.

11.10

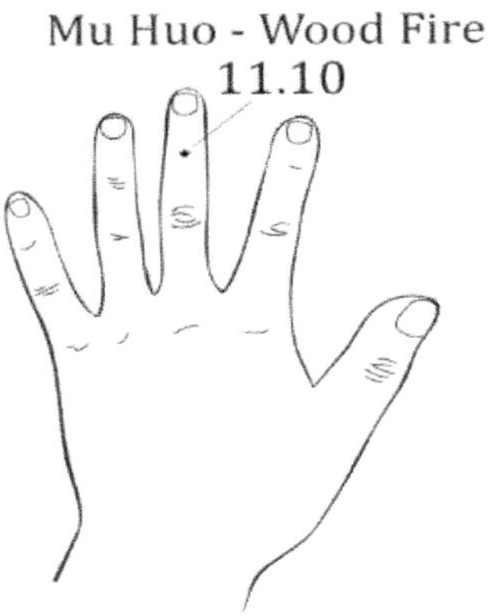

Indication: Hemiplegia, arm paralysis.

Location: In the center of the third finger crease of the middle finger on the dorsal side. Insert the needle obliquely in the direction of the little finger.

11.11

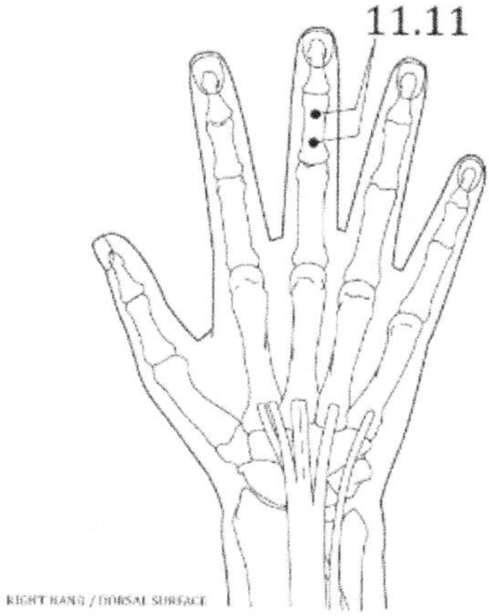

Fei Xin - Lung Heart

Indications: Pain on the spine, sacral vertebral pain, lumbar pain, neck pain, and calf pain originating in the spine.

Reaction areas: Heart, Lung

Location: On the middle segment of the dorsal aspect of the middle finger. Pinch the skin away from the bone, so you have access to more skin. Needle across the bone superficially, towards the little finger.

11.12

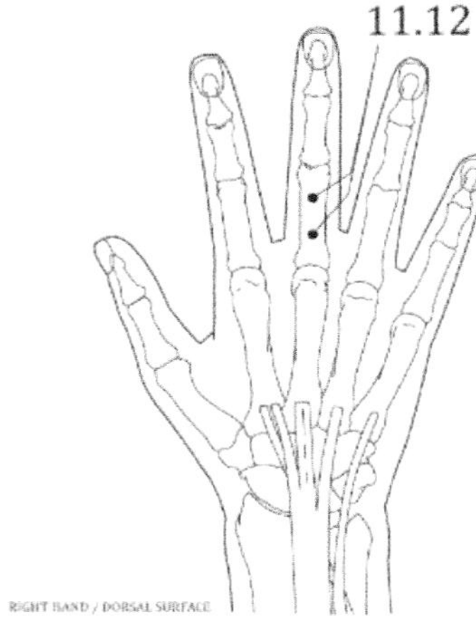

Er Jiao Ming - Two Corners Bright

Indications: Sprain in the lumbar region, pain in the supraorbital bone, nasal bone pain, kidney pain, nosebleeds, frontal headaches, eye issues – they brighten the eyes, glaucoma, intraocular eye pressure, and headaches from eye pressure. Other eye indications include, but are not limited to, macular degeneration, vision issues, and floaters.

Reaction areas: Kidney, Eyes

Location: On the midline of the proximal segment of the middle finger on the dorsal side.

11.13

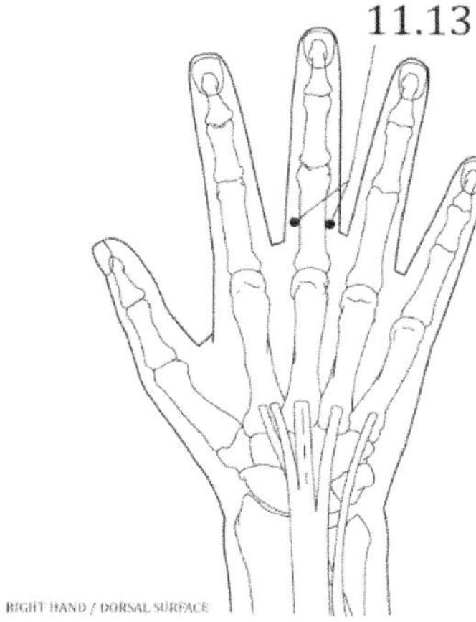

Dan - Gall Bladder

Indications: Child nightmares, night crying of children, knee pain, and gallbladder dysfunction.

Reaction area: Gallbladder

Location: In the middle of the proximal segment of the middle finger on the dorsal side. Insertion is .1 to .2 cun deep.

11.14

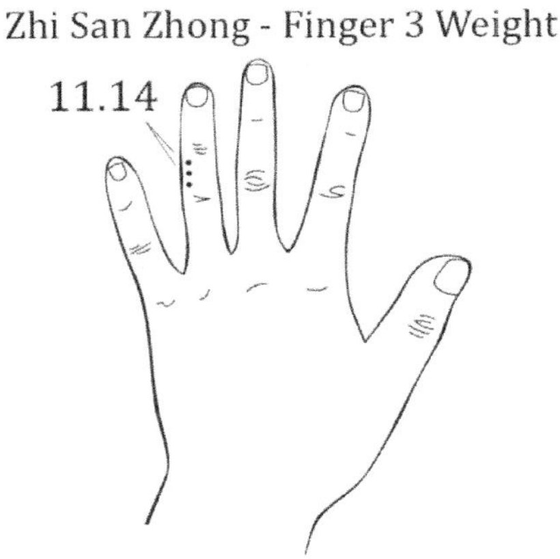

Indications: Facial paralysis, Bell's palsy, swollen breasts, muscle atrophy.

Location: On the dorsal side of the ring finger, on the ulnar side.

11.15

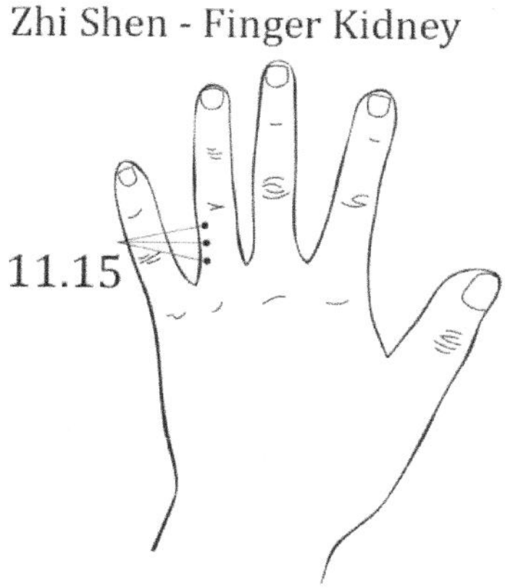

Indications: Kidney deficiency, thirst, heart deficiency, and back pain.

Location: On the dorsal side of the ring finger, on the ulnar side and proximal section.

11.16

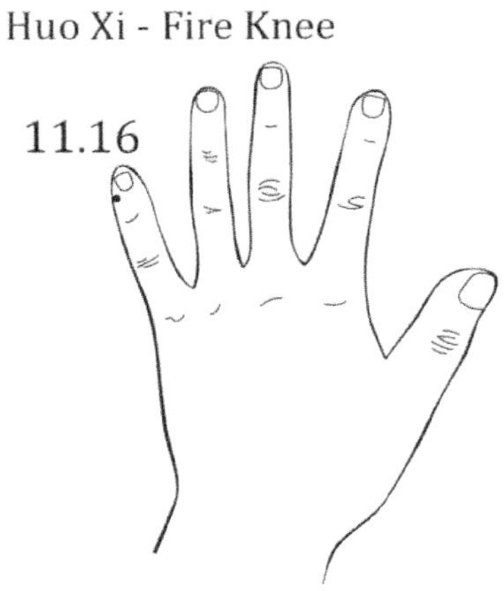

Indications: Knee pain, rheumatic heart disease, and arthritis.

Location: On the little finger, .2 cun lateral to the edge of the fingernail.

11.17

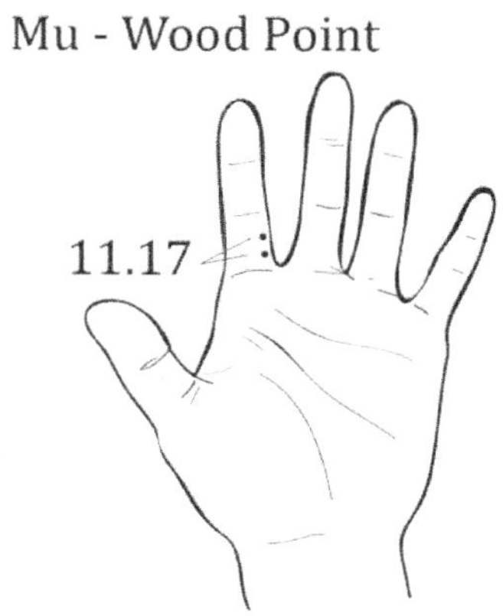

Indications: Liver Fire, irritability, dry eyes, dry nose, dermatitis of the hands, common cold, stress, anger, crying, stuffy congested nose, sinus issues, respiratory problems, urinary and genital issues, cystitis and hernia. Sweating of the hands.

Reaction area: Liver

Location: On the medial aspect of the index finger on the palmar side of the line of 0.2 cun away from the midline.

11.18

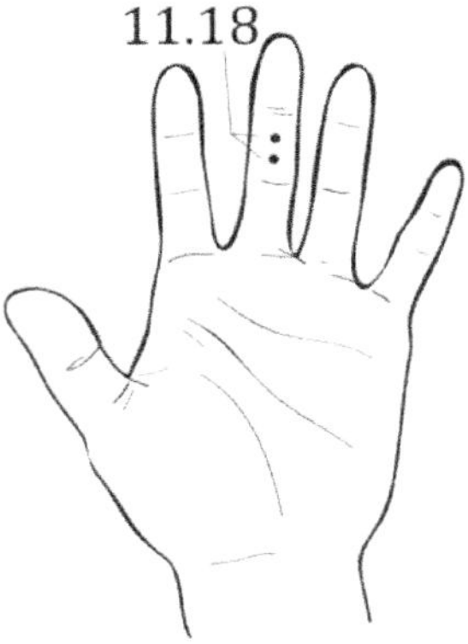

Indications: Spleen conditions such as spleen enlargement and inflammation.

Location: On the middle finger, palmar side, on the middle joint.

11.19

Xin Chang - Heart Normal

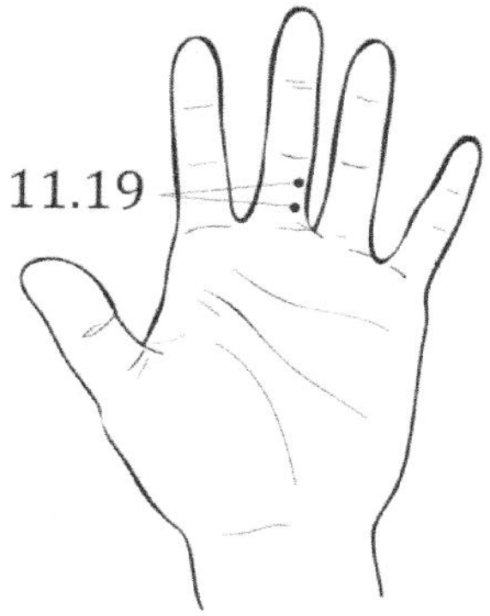

Indications: Palpitations, and heart disease.

Location: On the middle finger, ulnar side, on the midline of the proximal section. Insertion is .02 cun.

11.20

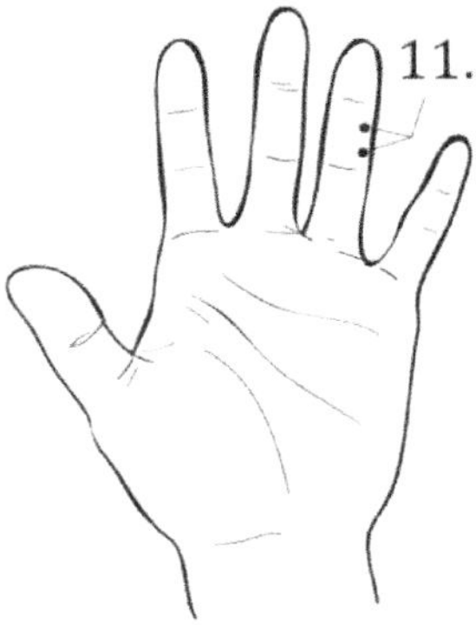

Indications: Hepatitis, cirrhosis, and swollen liver.

Location: On the ring finger, ulnar side of the palm.

11.21

San Yan - Three Eyes

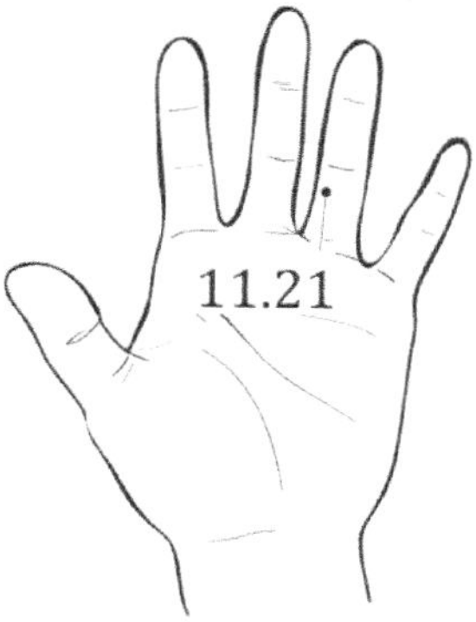

Indications: Functions similar to Stomach 36.

Location: On the ring finger, palmar side, radial side, .2 cun from the proximal crease. Insertion is .2 to .3 cun.

11.22

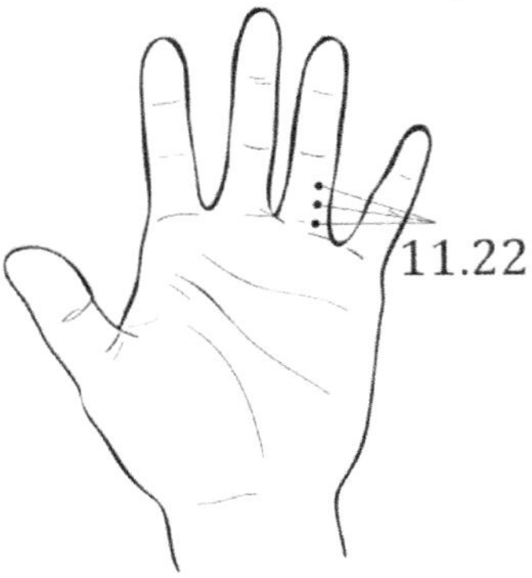

Indications: Bone enlargement, osteoarthritis.

Location: On the ring finger, ulnar and palmar side, on the proximal section. Insertion is .2 to .3 cun.

11.23

Yan Huang - Eye Yellow

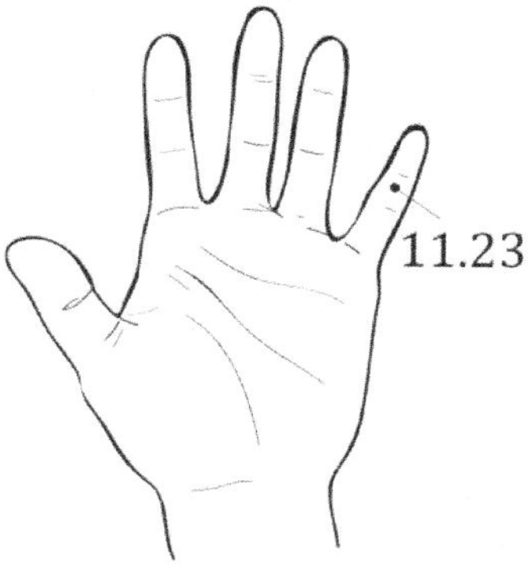

Indications: Conjunctival Icterus, which is yellow conjunctiva caused by jaundice.

Location: On the palmar side of the little finger, in the center of the middle segment of the finger joint.

11.24

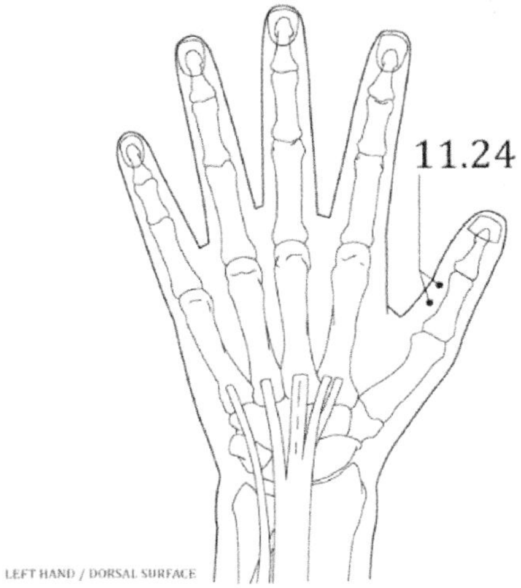

Fu Ke - Gynecology

Indications: Uterine inflammation, acute or chronic pelvic pain, abdominal distention, female infertility, irregular menstruation, dysmenorrhea, scanty menstruation, fibroids, change the position of the uterus during or after pregnancy, move blood, and or resolve uterine stagnation.

Reaction area: Uterus

Location: On the ulnar side of the dorsal, proximal segment of the thumb.

11.25

Zhi Yan - Stop Drooling

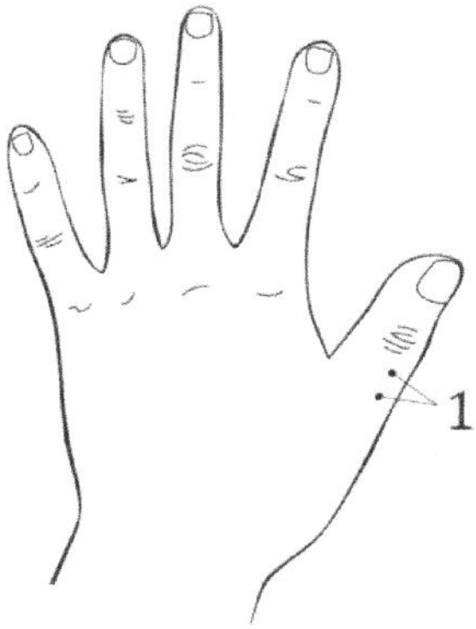

Indications: Drooling and slobbering in children

Location: On the radial, dorsal side on the proximal section of the thumb. Insertion is close to the bone at .1 to .2 cun.

11.26

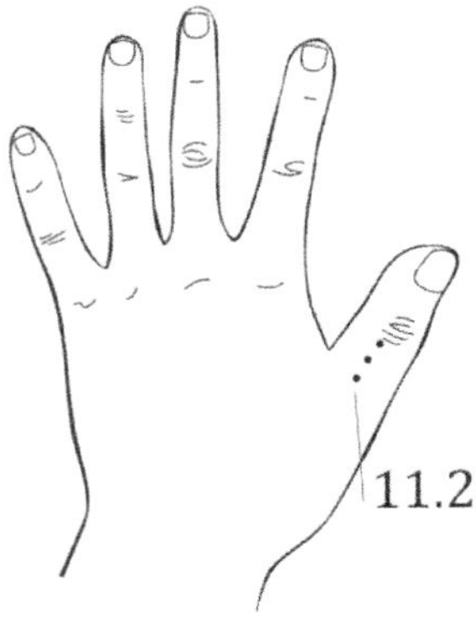

Indications: Delayed wound healing, abscesses, non-healing of wounds after surgery.

Location: On the dorsal side of the thumb, on the midline of the proximal section.

11.27

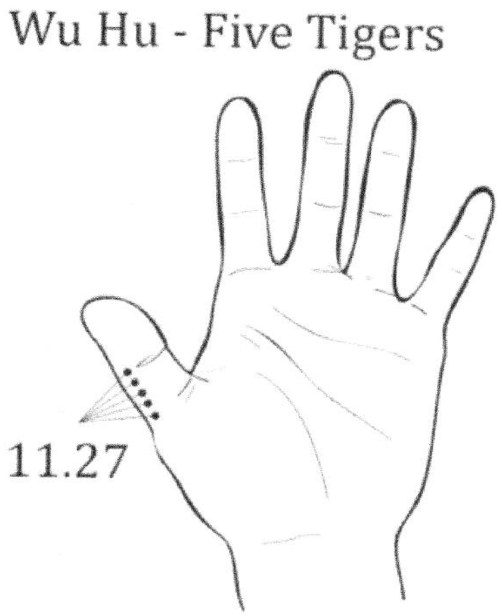

Indications: Swollen, achy joints, toe pain, gout, sore throat, swollen glands, pneumonia, cough, scrofula.

Reaction area: Spleen

Location: On the radial side of the proximal segment of the palmar side of the thumb.

22.01

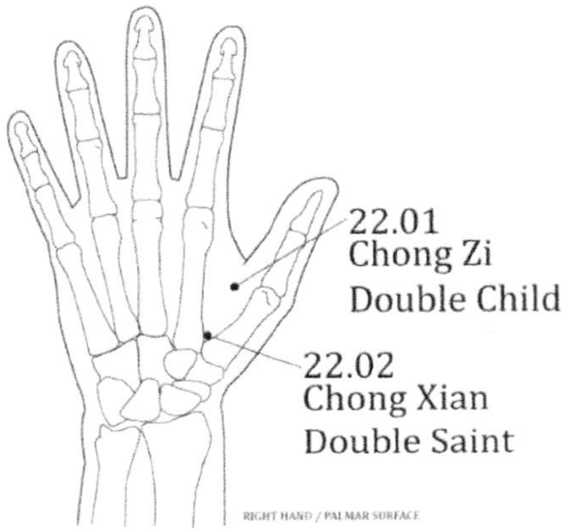

Indications: Back pain, pneumonia, cold and flu, cough, asthma, fibroids, and chest pain.

Reaction area: Lung

Location: On the palmar side of the hand, on the thenar eminence, about 1 cun distal to the skin fold, between the first and second metacarpals. Perpendicular insertion.

22.02

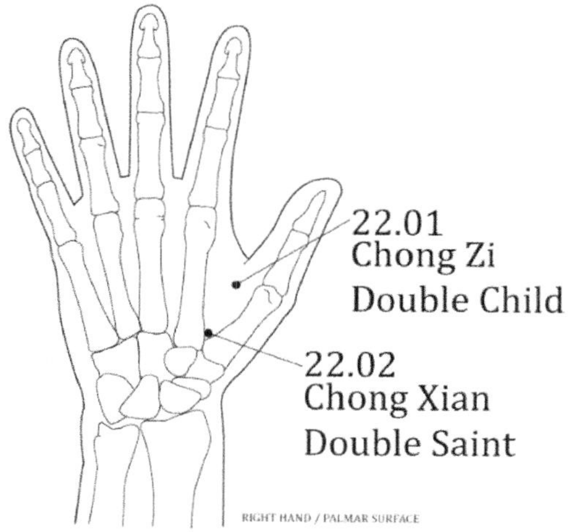

Indications: Back pain, pneumonia, cold and flu, cough, asthma, fibroids, chest pain, fever, palpitations, knee pain, and neck pain.

Reaction areas: Lung, Heart

Location: On the palmar side of the hand, between the first and second metacarpal bones, 2 cun from the skin fold.

22.03

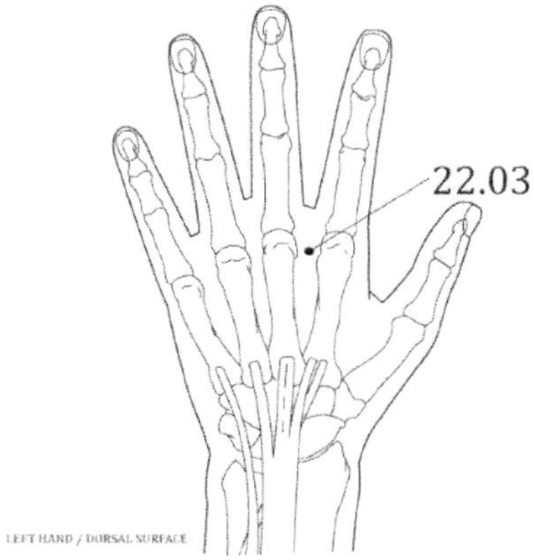

Shang Bai - Upper White

Indications: Eye diseases, sciatica, conjunctivitis, and heart pain.

Location: Between the MCP joints of the index and middle finger, .5 cun proximal.

22.04

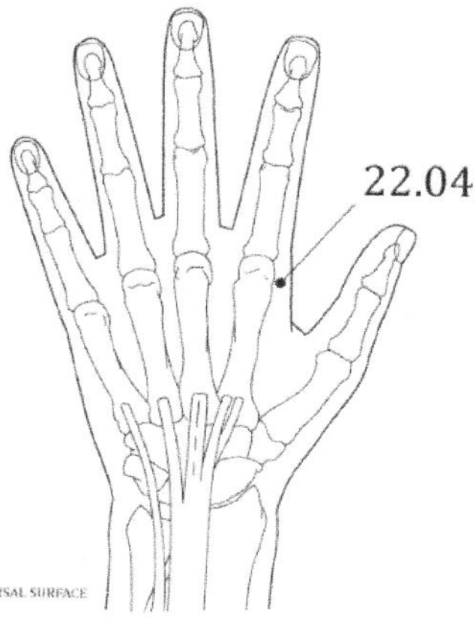

Da Bai - Big White

Indications: Childhood asthma, high fever in children (very effective) and sciatica due to lung deficiency.

Reaction area: Lung

Location: On the dorsum of the hand, the point is located in the depression 0.5 cun from the joint of the index finger and thumb, or between the first and second metacarpal bones. Contraindicated in pregnancy.

22.05

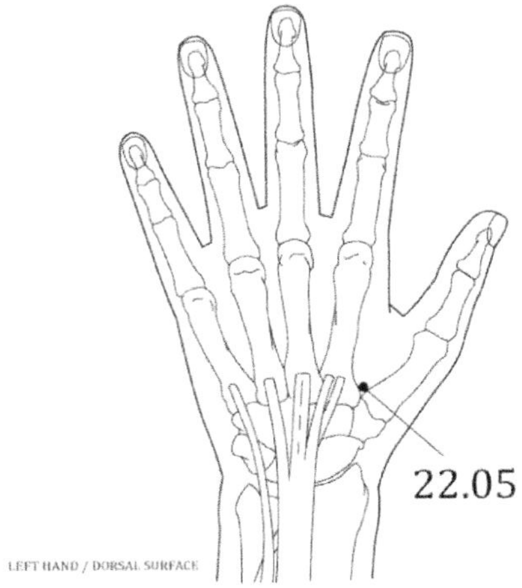

Ling Gu - Miraculous Bone

22.05, Ling Gu, is also called Spirit Bone

Indications: Sciatica, lower back pain, foot pain, Bell's palsy, hemiplegia, enlargement of bones, irregular menstruation, amenorrhea, difficult labor, back pain, tinnitus, migraine, dysmenorrhea, intestinal pain, dizziness, and a distending sensation of the head.

Reaction area: Lung

Location: Located in the junction between the index finger and thumb, the 1st and 2nd metacarpal bones, 1.2 cun from Da Bai (22.04), and directly opposite Chong Xian (22.02). Contraindicated in pregnancy.

22.06

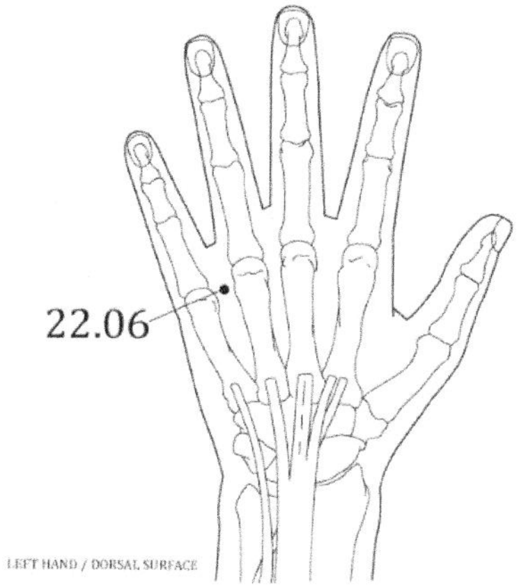

Zhong Bai - Center White

Indications: Lower back pain and sciatica due to kidney deficiency, back pain, dizziness, astigmatism, fatigue, lateral malleolus pain, and edema.

Reaction areas: Kidney, Heart, Spleen

Location: Located between the dorsal metacarpal bones of the little and ring fingers, 0.5 cun proximal to the metacarpophalangeal joint. 22.06 is commonly combined with 22.07.

22.07

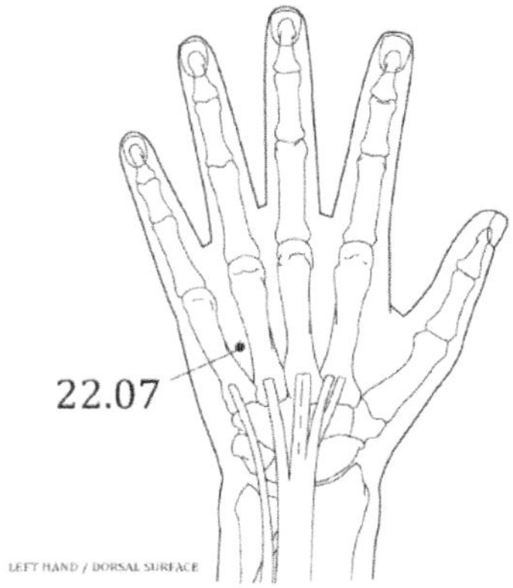

Xia Bai - Lower White

Indications: Toothache, slight liver pain. This point has the same indications as 22.06. Eye problems, lower back pain, tinnitus, dizziness, edema of the limbs, hypertension, heart palpitations, pain upon sitting or standing, pain in the chest that goes through to the back, blurred vision, fatigue, and headaches.

Reaction areas: Kidney, Heart, Spleen

Location: Located between the dorsal 4th and 5th metacarpal bones, 1.5 cun proximal to the metacarpophalangeal joint, 1 cun posterior to 22.06 on the dorsal side. Points 22.06 and 22.07 are commonly used together.

22.08

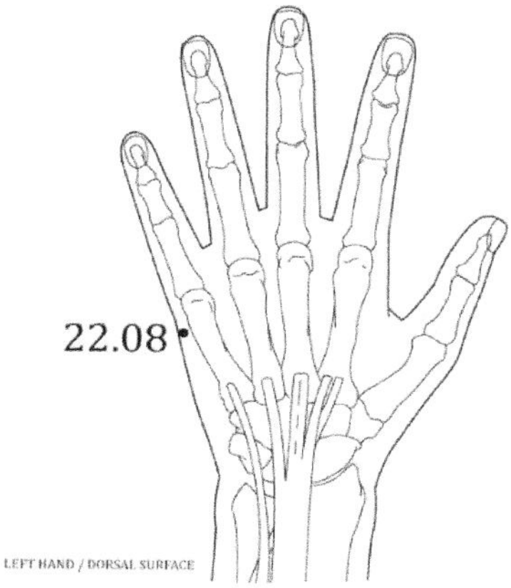

Wan Shun Yi - Wrist Flow, One

Indications: Headache, blurred vision, sciatica due to kidney deficiency, nephritis, edema of the limbs, heaviness and pain on both sides of the lower back, and back pain.

Reaction area: Kidney

Location: Located on the lateral side of the dorsal 5th metacarpal bone, 2.5 cun distal to the wrist crease. This point is always usually combined with with 22.09. Needle on one side only.

22.09

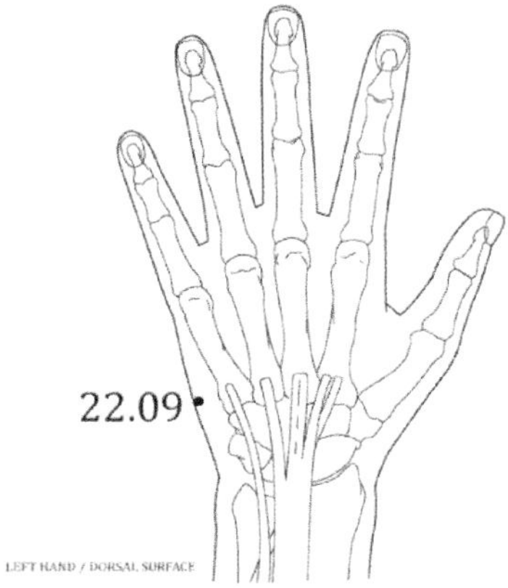

Wan Shun Er - Wrist Flow, Two

Indications: Headaches, nosebleed, blurred vision, and fatigue, sciatica due to kidney deficiency, edema, nephritis, swollen joints, lower back pain, spinal pain, and pain behind the knee, eye tics, trigeminal neuralgia, and sciatica on the BL channel, toothaches, eye pain, tinnitus, and lower abdominal distension.

Reaction area: Kidney

Location: Located on the dorsal side of the lateral side of the 5th metacarpal bone, 1.5 cun distal to the wrist crease. It is 1 cun posterior to 22.08. Insertion is 1 to 1.5 cun. Combine with 22.08.

22.10

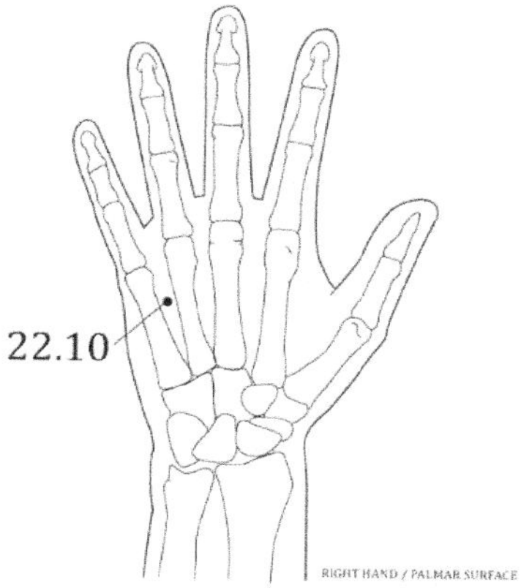

Shou Jie - Hand Release

Indications: Fainting from needle shock, and stabbing pain.

Location: At the TCM point Heart 8, where the tip of the little finger touches the palm when a fist is formed.

22.11

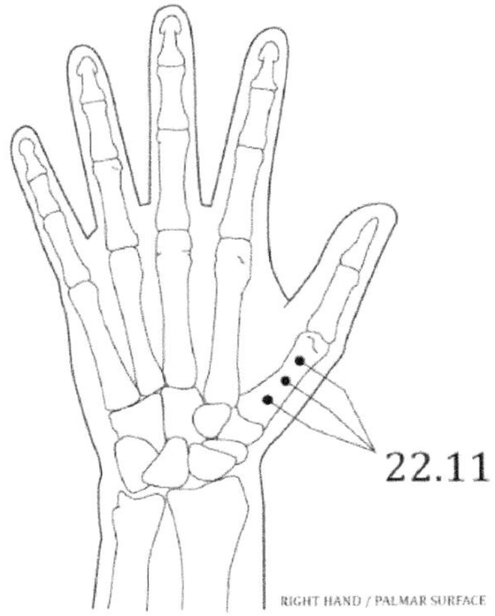

Tu Shui - Earth Water

Indications: Gastritis, chronic stomach disease, and gastric ulcer.

Reaction areas: Kidney, Spleen

Location: On the palmar side of the first metacarpal bone, on the radial side.

33.01, 33.02, 33.03

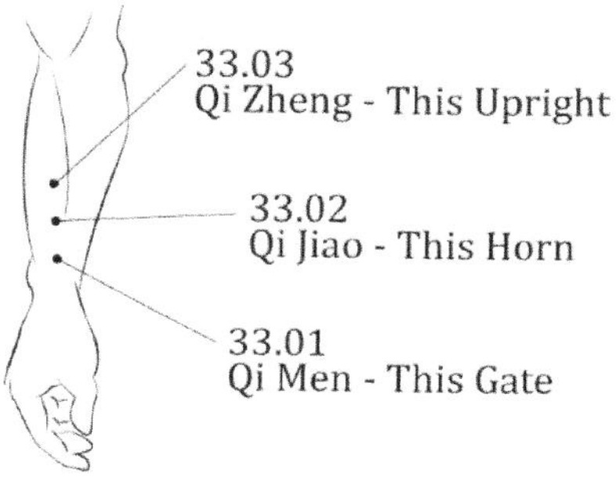

Indications: Irregular menstruation, reddish leukorrhea, rectal prolapse, and hemorrhoid pain.

Reaction area: Lung

Location: This point is located on the radial side of the forearm, on the line between LI 5 and LI 11. Point 33.01 is located two cun from the wrist crease. Point 33.02 is two cun proximal to 33.01, 33.03 is two cun proximal to 33.02. Points 33.01, 33.02, and 33.03 are always used together.

33.04, 33.05, 33.06

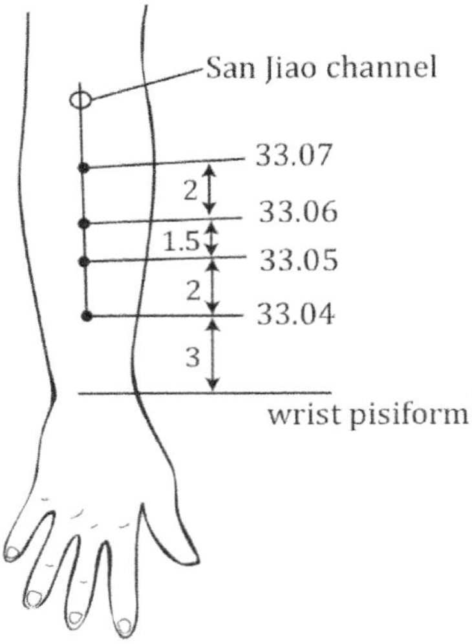

33.04, Huo Chuan, Fire Threaded

Indications: Constipation, forearm pain, and palpitations.

Reaction areas: Lung, Heart (for all four points.)

Location: This point is the same as TCM point SJ 6. It is 3 cun from the wrist crease. Insertion for all points on this Dao Ma is .5 to 1.5 cun.

33.04, 33.05, 33.06

33.05, Huo Ling, Fire Mound

Indications: Chest oppression and pain, hand cramps, carpal tunnel syndrome, and finger nerve issues.

Location: 2 cun proximal to 33.04.

33.06, Huo Shan, Fire Mountain

Indications: Chest stuffiness, and hand cramps.

Location: 1.5 cun proximal to 33.05.

These points are a Dao Ma. Dr. Maher translates them as "Hold Three Fires." Dr. Chuan Min-Wang translates them as "Upper Three Fires Warm the Body." Dr. Maher uses a different numbering system from other teachers. This Dao Ma is numbered as 33-11 in his book *Advanced Tung Style Acupuncture: The Dao Ma Needling Technique.*

33.07

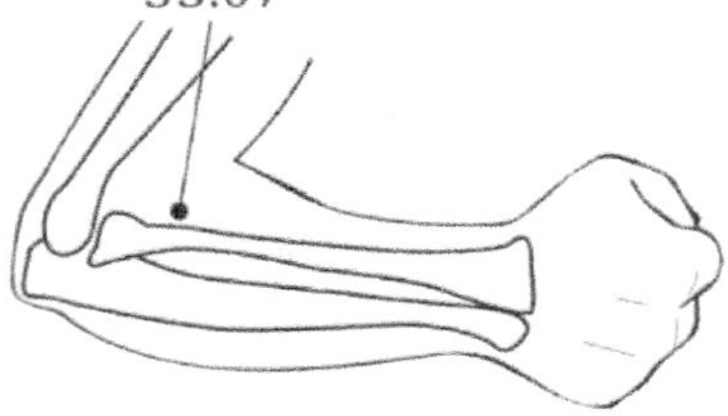

Indications: Coughing, asthma, common cold, allergies, sinusitis, sciatica, lower back and leg pain, fatigue, dizziness, blurred vision, and eye strain.

Location: This point is the same as TCM point LI 10. 2 cun proximal to 33.06.

33.08, 33.09

Two Metal Dao Ma

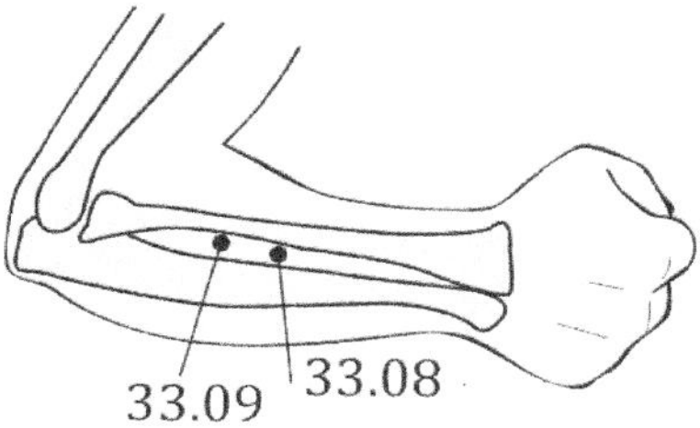

33.08, Shou Wu Jin, Arm Five Metal

33.09, Shou Qian Jin, Arm 1000 Metal

Indications: Sciatica, abdominal pain, leg pain, foot pain and numbness.

Reaction area of 33.08: Lung
Reaction area of 33.09: Liver

33.08, 33.09

Location: Perpendicular insertion 5 fen lateral to the TW channel, on the lateral side of the ulna.

Point 33.08 is 6.5 cun proximal from the wrist crease
Point 33.09 is 8.0 cun proximal from the wrist crease
Point 33.09 is also measured as 1.5 cun proximal to 33.08.

33.10

Three Gates Dao Ma, 33.10, 33.11, 33.12

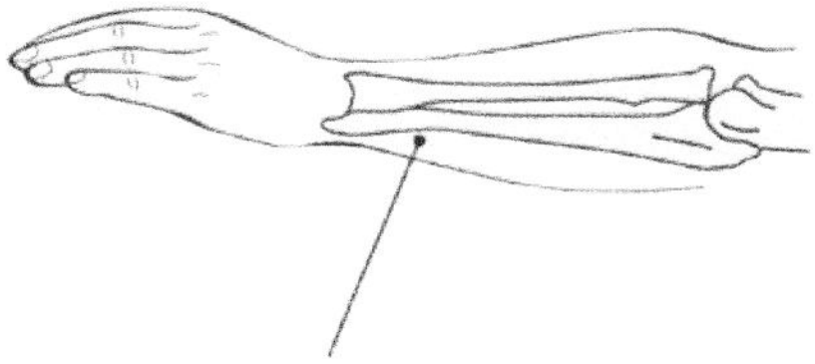

33.10

Chang Men - Intestine Gate

Indications: Enteritis caused by hepatitis, dizziness, blurred vision, abdominal pain, diarrhea.

Reaction areas: Liver, Kidney

Location: Located on the medial side of the ulna on the SI channel, three cun proximal to the pisiform bone. Insertion is 0.3-0.5 cun deep. Points 33.10, 33.11, and 33.12 are usually used together as a Dao Ma.

33.10, 33.11, and 33.12

Three Gates Dao Ma

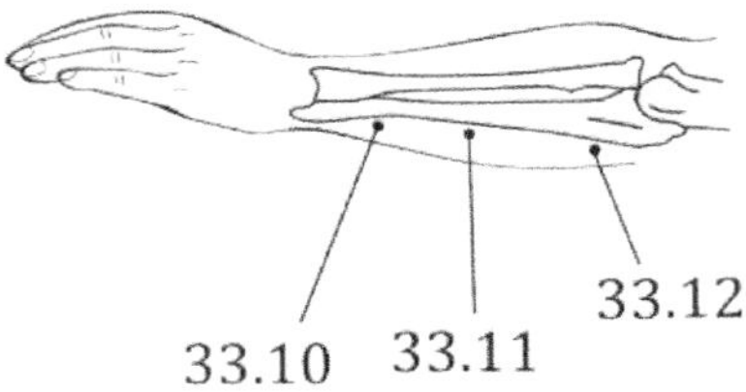

33.11

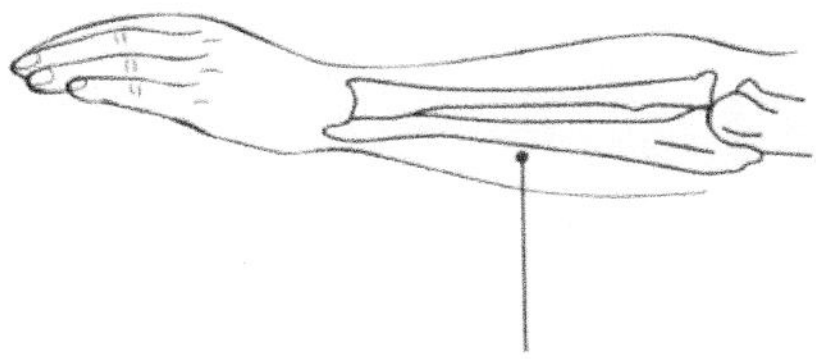

33.11
Gan Men - Liver Gate

Indication: Acute hepatitis.

Reaction area: Liver

Location: On the ulnar side on the SI channel, 6 cun proximal to the pisiform bone.

33.12

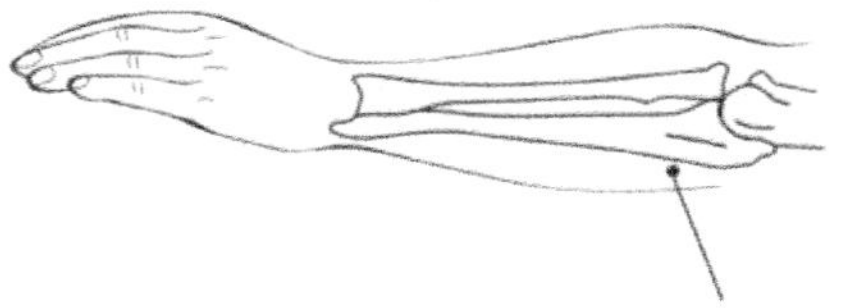

Xin Men - Heart Gate

Indications: Heart inflammation, palpitations, suffocating feeling in the chest, vomiting, and dry cholera. Liver fire, medial knee pain, coccyx pain, groin pain, medial thigh pain, sciatica, and sacral pain.

Reaction area: Heart

Location: Located in the depression on the medial side of the inferior ulna, 1.5 cun distal to the elbow. It is contraindicated to needle this point bilaterally.

33.13, 33.14, 33.15

Three Scholars Dao Ma

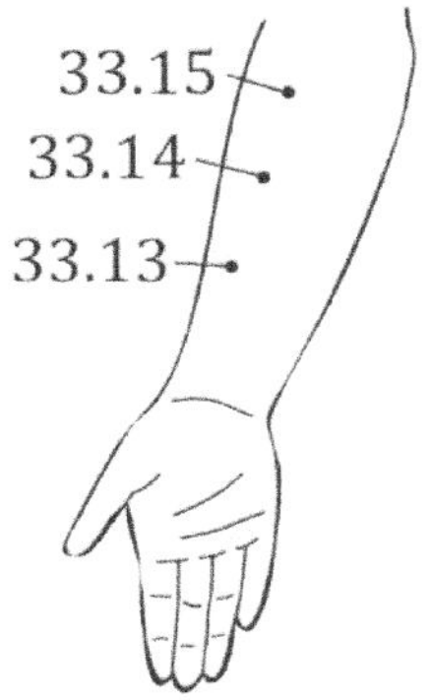

33.13, Ren Shi, Humanity Scholar
33.14, Di Shi, Earth Scholar
33.15, Tian Shi, Heavenly Scholar

Three Scholars Dao Ma

Indications: Asthma, rhinitis, arm pain, shoulder pain, palm pain, common cold, and suffocating sensation in the chest.

Reaction areas: Heart, Lung

Locations:
33.13 is on the Lung channel 4 cun above the lateral side of the radius.

33.13, 33.14, 33.15

Three Scholars Dao Ma

33.14 is on the Lung channel 7 cun above the wrist crease.
33.15 in on the Lung channel 10 cun above the wrist crease. It is located at Lung 6.

Insertion is 1 to 1.5 cun.

33.16

Qu Ling - Curved Mound

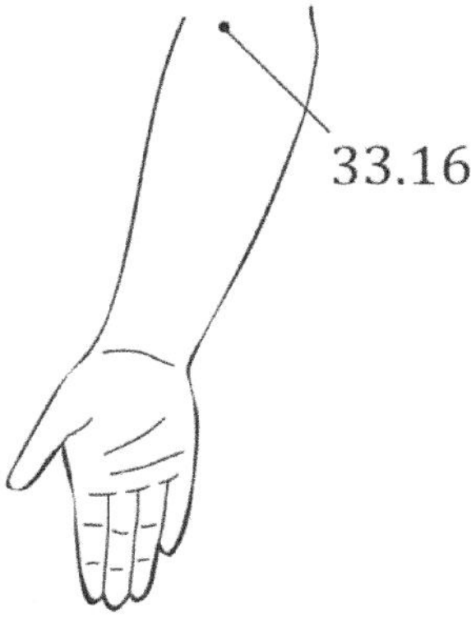

Indications: Muscle spasms, digestive issues, elbow pain, asthma, heart palpitations.

Reaction areas: Heart and Lungs

Location: In the center of the cubital fossa crease, on the radial side of the biceps tendon.

44.01

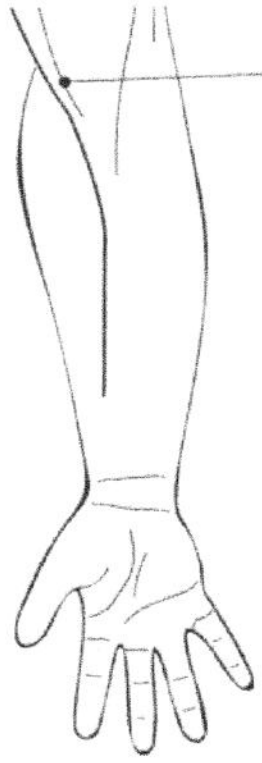

Indications: Common cold, laryngitis, allergies.

Location: 1.5 cun proximal to the cubital fossa, on the anterior side of the humerus bone. Insertion is .5 to an inch.

44.02, 44.03

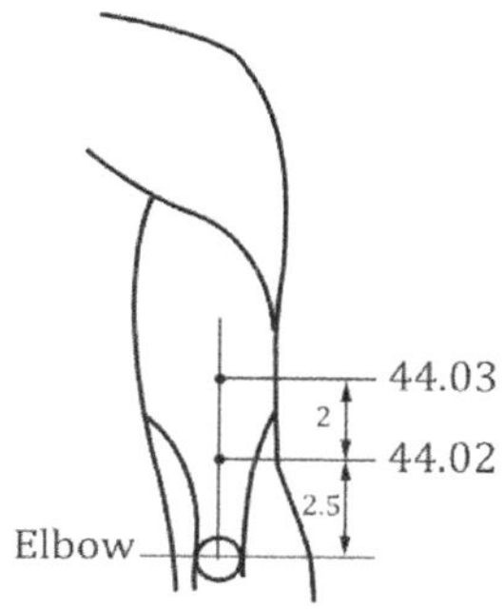

44.02, Hou Zhui, Back Vertebra
44.03, Shou Ying, Head Wisdom

Indications: Dislocation and distending pain of the vertebrae, nephritis, hypertension, and lower back pain.

Reaction areas: Liver, Heart, Spine

Locations: For best results some sources say to touch the bone.

44.02 – Located on the posterior side of the humerus, 2.5 cun above the cubital crease on the Triple Warmer channel.
44.03 – Located on the posterior side of the humerus, 4.5 cun above the cubital crease on the Triple Warmer channel. It is 2 cun above 44.02.

44.04

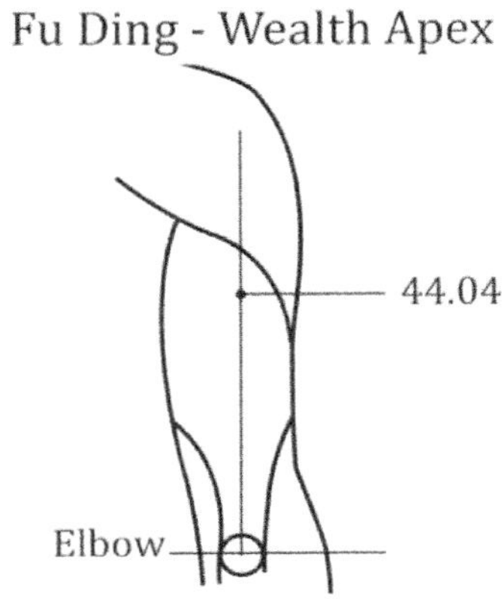

Indications: Hypertension, fatigue, dizziness, headache.

Reaction area: Heart

Location: On the posterior side of the humerus. 2.5 cun above 44.03, 7 cun from the cubital crease. Insertion is .3 to .5 cun.

Dr. Chuan-Min Wang combines 44.04 and 44.05 and calls it the "Buster of Hypertension."

44.05

Hou Zhi - Back Branch

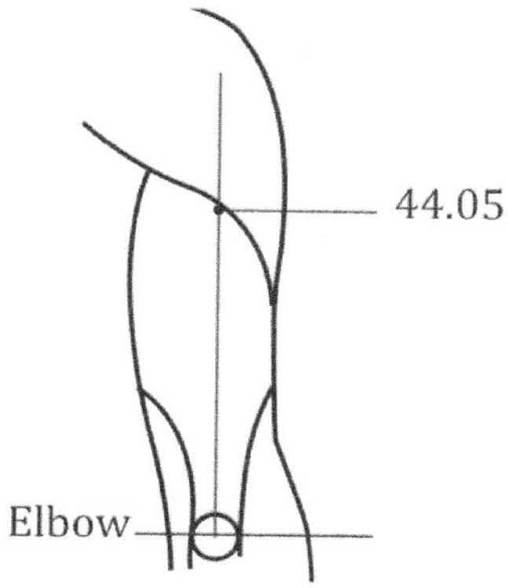

Indications: Hypertension, dizziness, headache, neck pain, facial paralysis.

Reaction area: Heart

Location: 1 cun from 44.04, 8 cun above the cubital crease. Often combined with 44.04. Insertion is .3 to .7 cun.

44.06

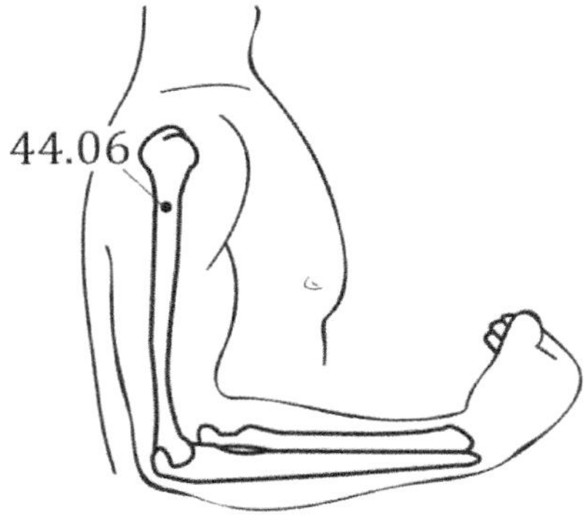

Jian Zhong - Shoulder Center

Indications: Knee pain, skin diseases, polio, hemiplegia, palpitations, arteriosclerosis, nosebleeds, and shoulder pain.

Reaction area: Heart

Location: On the lateral side of the humerus, 2.5 cun inferior to the acromion joint.

44.07

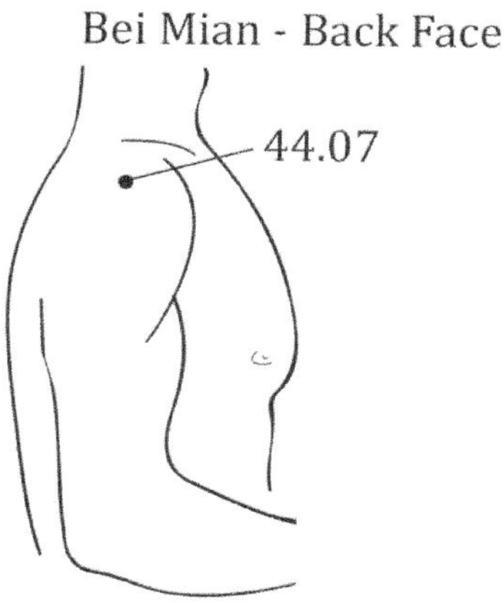

Indications: Regulates Lung Qi, abdominal distension, flatulence, weak voice, laryngitis, nausea, vomiting, acute enteritis, sciatica, and fatigue.

Location: In the center of the acromion joint, in the depression when arm is raised. Insertion is 0.3-0.5 cun deep. In the area of Large Intestine 15.

44.08

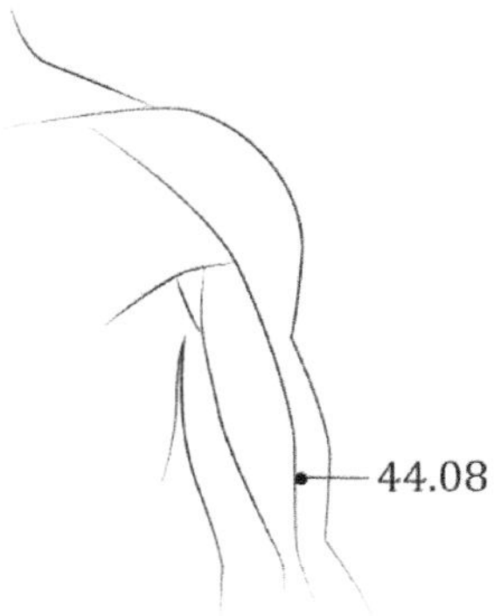

Ren Zong - Human Ancestor

Indications: Foot pain, lower leg pain, elbow or arm pain, jaundice, edema, spleen enlargement, common cold, asthma.

Location: In the depression between the lateral border of the humerus and biceps brachii, 3 cun superior to the cubital crease. Insertion is .8 cun. This point is always combined with 44.09 and 44.10.

Points 44.08, 44.09, and 44.10 are combined into a Dao Ma. Dr. Maher calls this “Brachial Three Ancestors.”

44.09

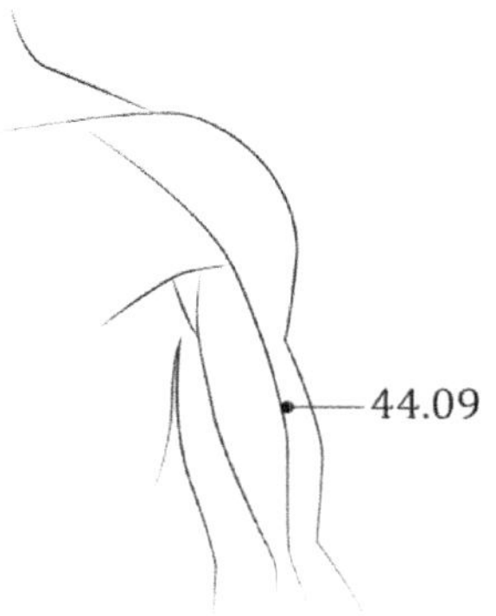

Di Zong - Earth Ancestor

Indications: Yang collapse, heart disease and arteriosclerosis

Location: 2 cun superior to 44.08, 6 cun above the cubital crease. Combine with 44.08 and 44.10.

44.10

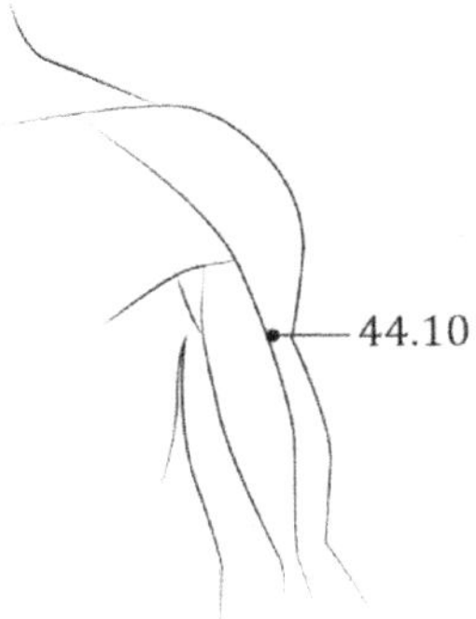

Tian Zong - Heavenly Ancestor

Indications: Post-polio syndrome, diabetes mellitus, leg pain, leucorrhea, body odor, vaginitis, urogenital pain, calf pain.

Reaction areas: Legs, Six Fu-bowels

Location: In the depression between the lateral side of the humerus and the posterior side of the biceps brachii muscle, 3 cun superior to 44.09. Insertion is 1 to 1.5 cun. Combine points 44.08, 44.09, and 44.10. Six cun above the elbow joint.

44.08, 44.09, 44.10

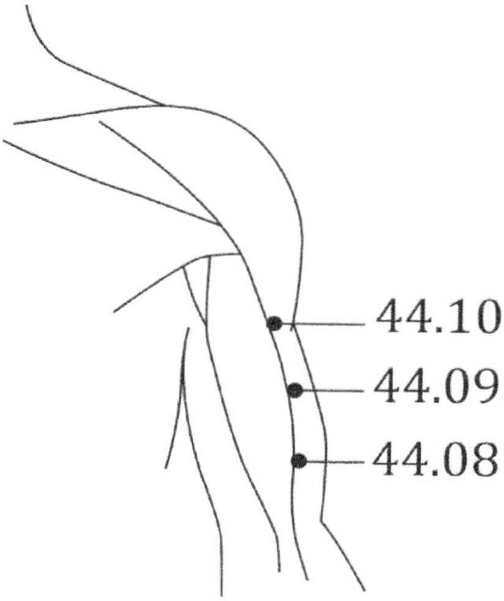

44.11

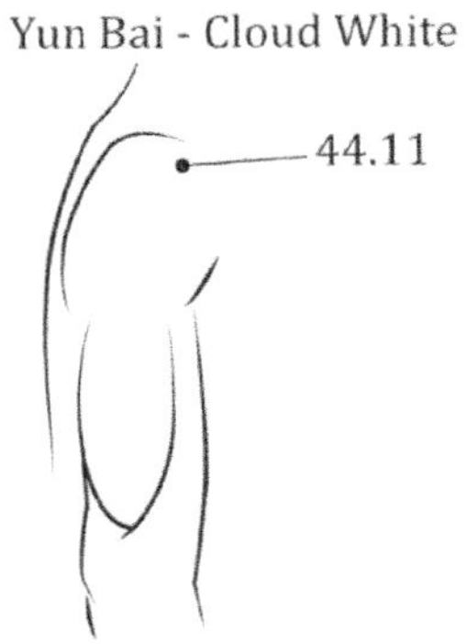

Indications : Vaginitis, vaginal pain, vaginal itching, red or white leucorrhea, post-polio syndrome.

Reaction areas : Lungs and six bowels.

Location: One cun anterior to 44.06. Insertion is .3 to .5 cun. Combine 44.11, and 44.12.

44.12

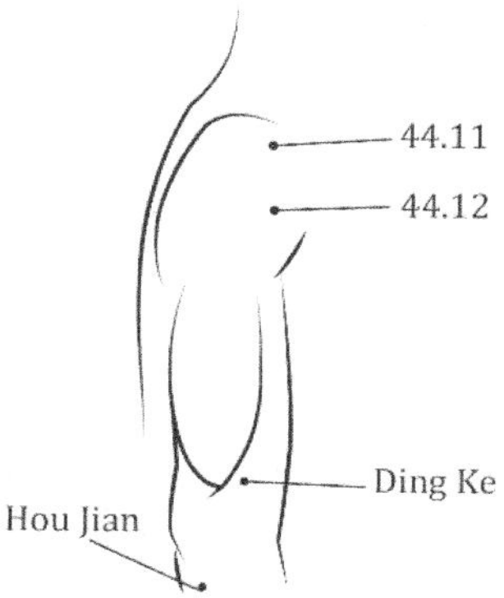

Indications: Armpit odor, calf pain, foot pain, post-polio syndrome.

Reaction areas: Kidneys, lungs.

Location: Two cun slightly anterior and inferior to 44.11. Insertion is .3 to .5 cun.

44.13

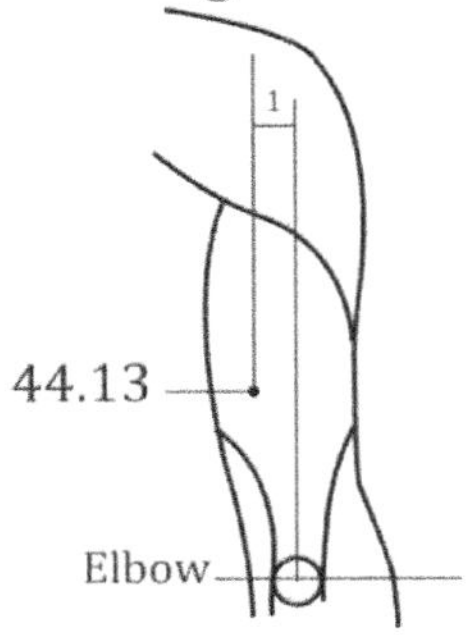

Indications: Hypertension, dizziness, lower back pain, and fatigue.

Location: On the posterior side of the upper arm, 1 cun posterior to 44.03. Insertion is .6 to 1 cun. Combine with 44.14. Located 4.5 cun above the elbow joint.

44.14

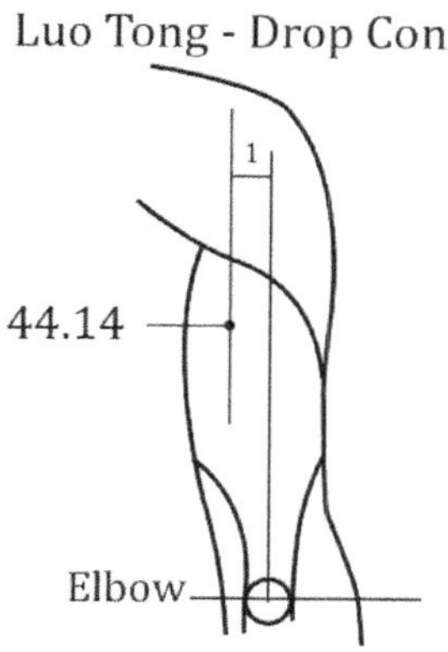

Indications: Hypertension, dizziness, fatigue, and lower back pain.

Location: On the posterior arm, 1 cun posterior to 44.04. Insertion is .5 to 1 cun. Combine with 44.08, 44.09, and 44.10. Located 7 cun above the elbow joint.

44.15

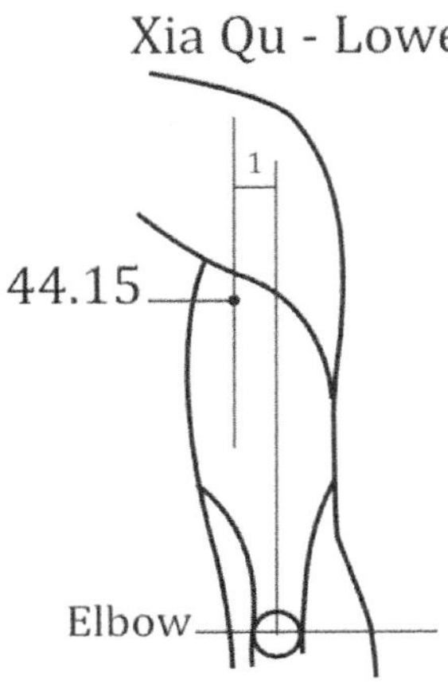

Indications: Hypertension, Post-polio syndrome, sciatica, hemiplegia.

Location: On the posterior side of the upper arm, 1 cun posterior to 44.05. Insertion is .6 to 1 cun.

44.16

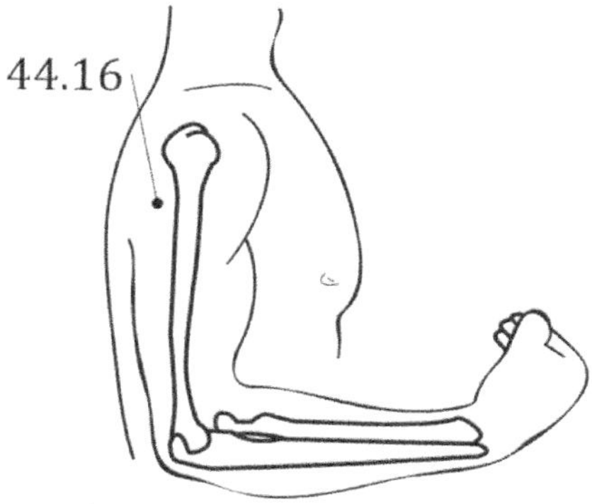

Shang Qu - Upper Curve

Indications: Sciatica, arm pain, leg pain, Post-polio syndrome, and hypertension.

Location: On the posterior side of the upper arm, 1 cun posterior to 44.06. Insertion is .6 to 1.5 cun. Located 3 cun below the acromion process.

44.17

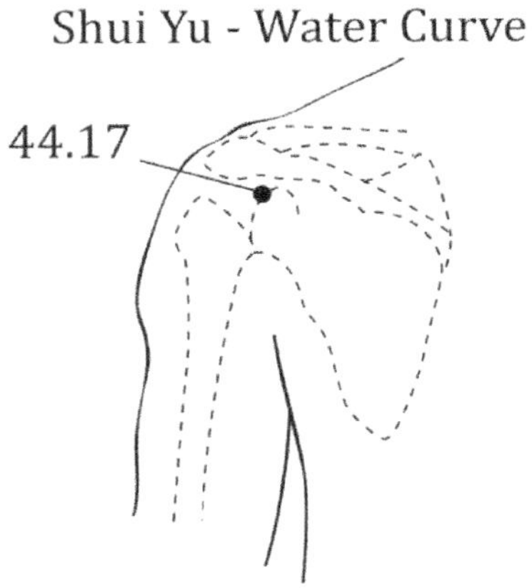

Indications: Lower back pain, kidney stones, nephritis, wrist pain, carpal tunnel syndrome, arm pain, leg muscle pain, general weakness. Treats kidney issues in general.

Location: On the posterior side of the upper arm, 2 cun posterior and inferior to 44.07. Located 2 cun below the acromion process. Located at Small Intestine 10. Insertion is .3 to .5 cun.

55.01

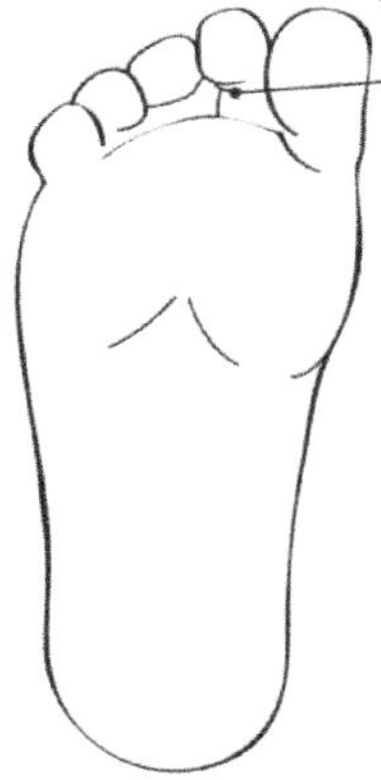

Indications: Difficult labor, retention of placenta, angina.

Location: On the plantar side of the second toe, in the center of the distal crease. This point can be bled.

55.02

Hua Gu Yi - Flower Bone One

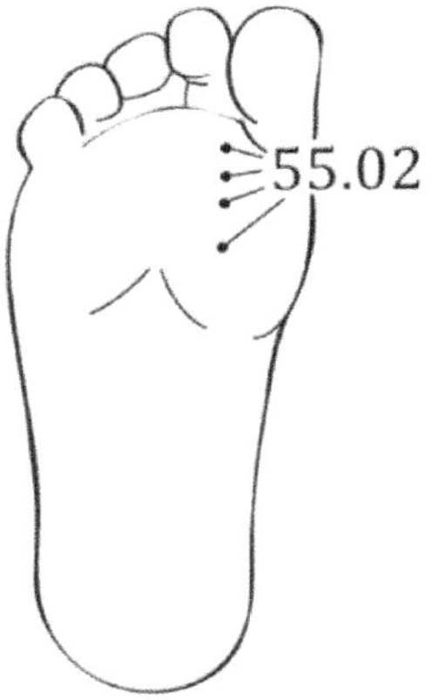

Indications: Trachoma, which is a bacterial infection of the eye caused by chlamydia. Blepharitis, which is inflammation of the eyelids, conjunctivitis, nasal pain, light sensitivity, tearing on exposure to the wind, headache, toothache, tinnitus, loss of hearing, pain of the nasal bone.

Reaction areas: Spleen, Lung, Kidney

Location: Between the 1st and 2nd metatarsal bones on the plantar surface. Insertion is up to 1 cun.

55.03

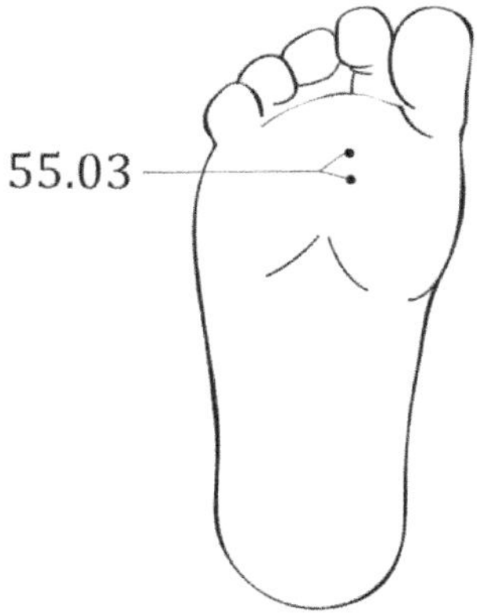

Indications: Finger weakness, arm pain that inhibits lifting.

Location: On the plantar surface, between the first and second metatarsal bones.

55.04

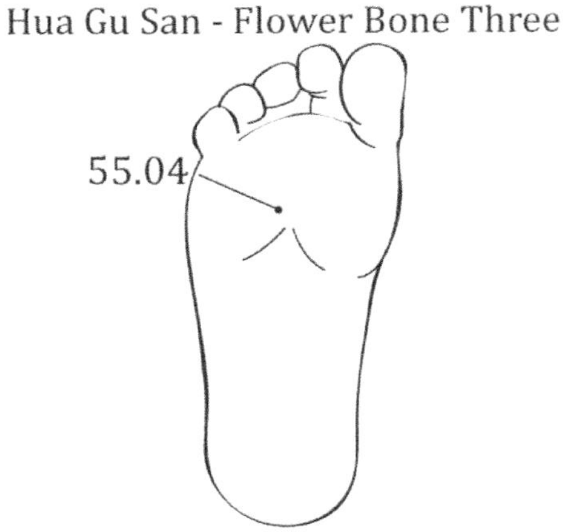

Indications: Back pain, spinal pain, leg and foot numbness, and sciatica.

Location: On the plantar side, between the third and fourth metatarsal bones.

55.05

Hua Gu Si - Flower Bone Four

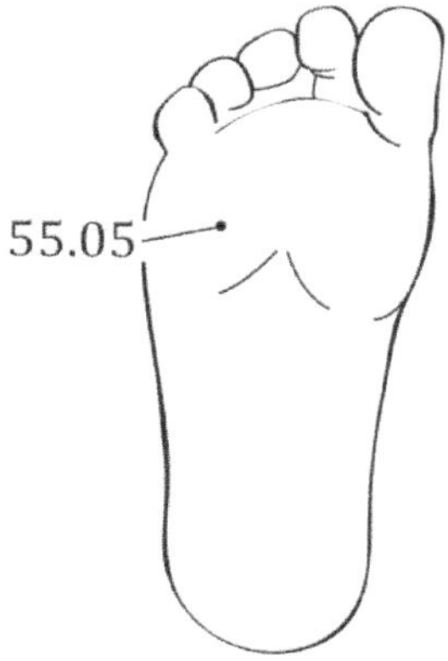

Indications: Pain on the spine, sciatica, stomach and abdominal pain, stops bleeding.

Location: Between the fourth and fifth metatarsal bones of the foot. Insertion is .5 to 1 cun deep. Located 1.5 cun posterior to the web between the fourth and fifth toes.

55.06

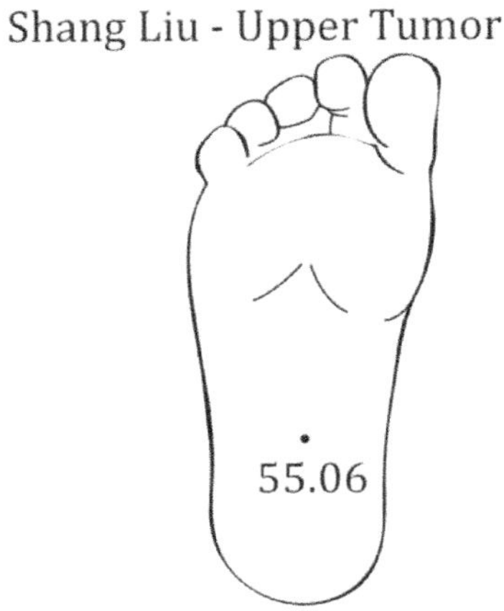

Indications: Brain tumor, headache, swelling of the cerebellum, trigeminal neuralgia, fatigue, nasal congestion, occipital pain, and nosebleed.

Reaction area: Brain

Location: Located in the center of the anterior edge of the heel.

66.01

Hai Bao - Sea Seal

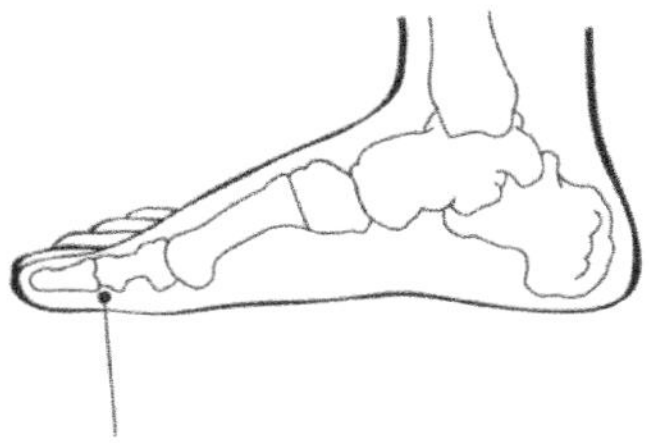

Indications: Hernia, conjunctivitis, pain in the eye canthus, vaginitis, pain of the thumb and index finger.

Location: In the middle of the big toe, anterior to Spleen 2. Insertion is .1 to .3 cun.

66.02

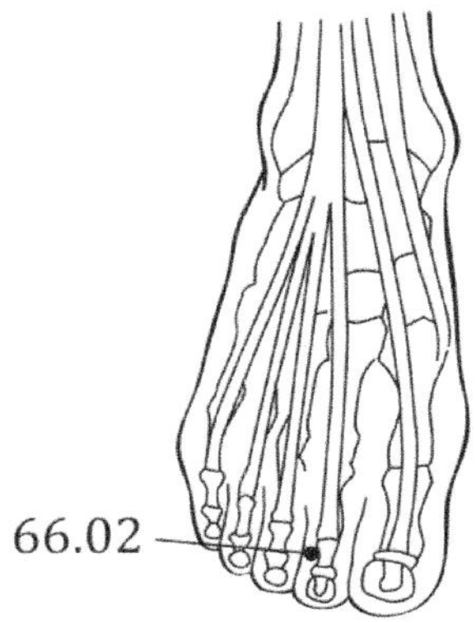

Mu Fu - Wood Wife

Indications: Reddish leukorrhea, irregular menstruation, dysmenorrhea, fallopian tube blockage, infertility.

Reaction area: Heart

Location: On the dorsal side of the second toe, .3 cun lateral to the center of the middle section. Insertion is .2 to .4 cun.

66.03

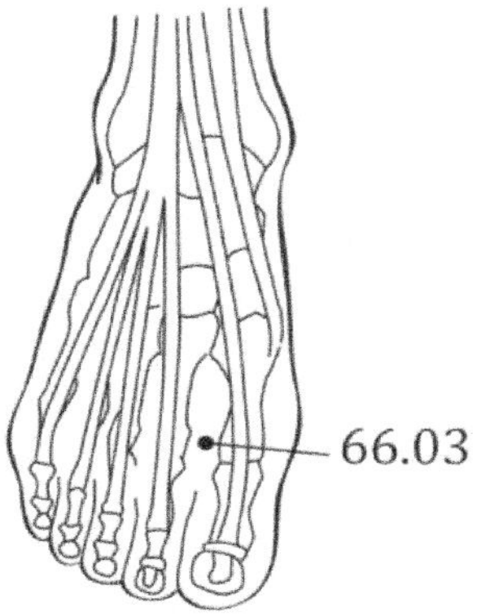

Huo Ying - Fire Hard

Indications: Strengthens the heart, an emergency point for fainting or heart attack. Palpitations, tumor of the uterus, uterine fibroids, retention of placenta, inflammation of the uterus, chin pain, pain of the temporomandibular joint (TMJ), grinding teeth from stress, and dizziness.

Reaction areas: Heart, Liver

Location: Between the 1st and 2nd metatarsal bones, 0.5 cun from the metatarsophalangeal joints, on the dorsal surface.

66.04

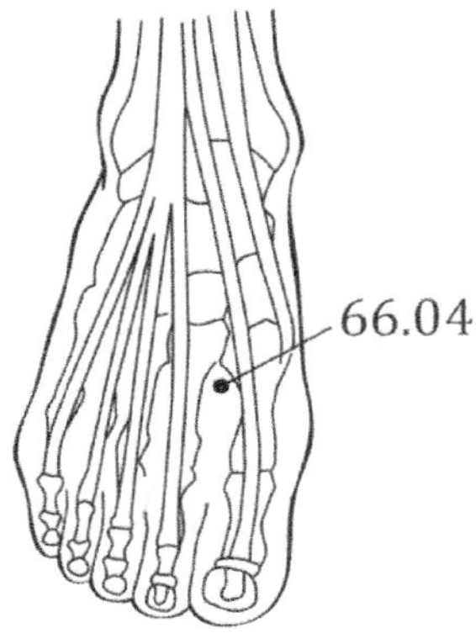

Huo Zhu - Fire Master

Indications: Emergency point for heart attacks, enlargement of the bones, headache, inflammation or tumors of the uterus, gastrointestinal diseases, liver diseases, exhaustion, breech presentation, pain in the hands and feet, difficult labor, headache due to heart problems, liver and stomach disease, inflammation and tumors of the uterus.

Reaction area: Heart

Location: One cun posterior to 66.03. Perpendicular insertion. This is as close to the juncture of the first and second metatarsal joint as possible.

66.05

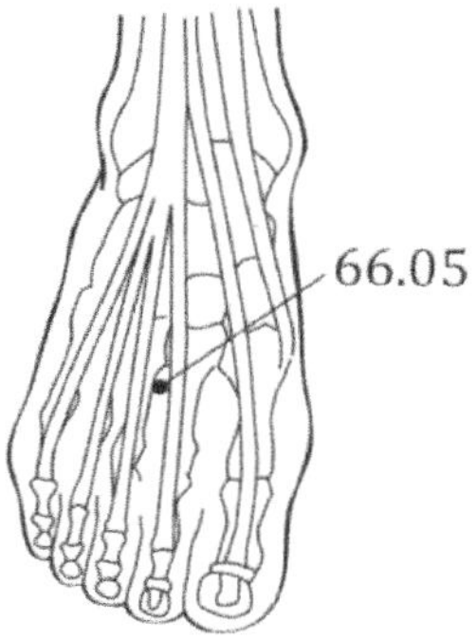

Men Jin - Gate Metal

Indications: Inflammation of small intestine, gastritis, abdominal distension, migraines, and appendicitis.

Reaction areas: Stomach, Intestines, Duodenum, Uterus

Location: This point is at the juncture of the 2nd and 3rd metatarsal bones, the tighter to the junction of the toes you can get the better the point works.

Do not treat bilaterally. Combine with ST 44 for rectal prolapse. Dr. Lee combines 66.05 and 77.09 for migraines. 66.05 can be bled to treat migraines.

66.06

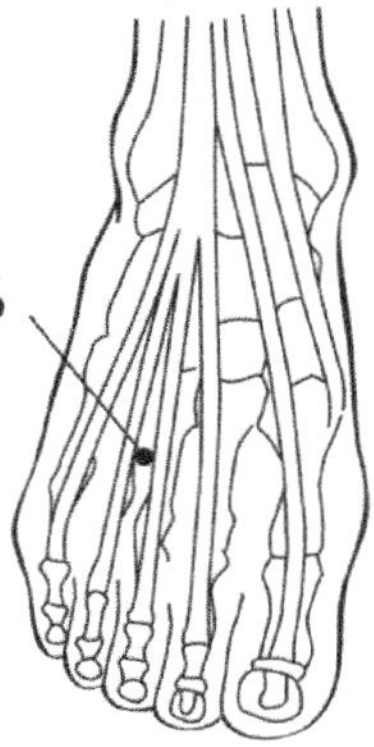

Mu Liu - Wood Remain

Indications: Spleen enlargement, liver disease, indigestion, gallbladder disorders such as gallstones, polio, fatigue, middle finger pain and stiffness, headache.

Reaction areas: Liver, Spleen

Location: Anterior to the junction of the third and fourth metatarsal bones, which is approximately 1.5 cun from the metatarsophalangeal joint. Insertion is 1 to 1.5 cun. This point can be combined with 66.07 for increased effectiveness.

66.07

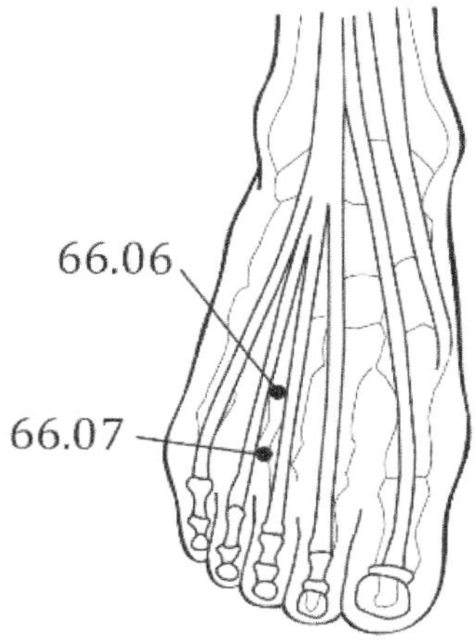

66.07, Mu Dou, Wood Dipper

Indications: Liver disease, indigestion, fatigue, gallbladder disease, polio, splenomegaly.

Reaction areas: Liver, Spleen

Location: Between the third and fourth metatarsal bones, .5 cun proximal to the metatarsophalangeal joint. Insertion is .5 to 1 cun.

66.08

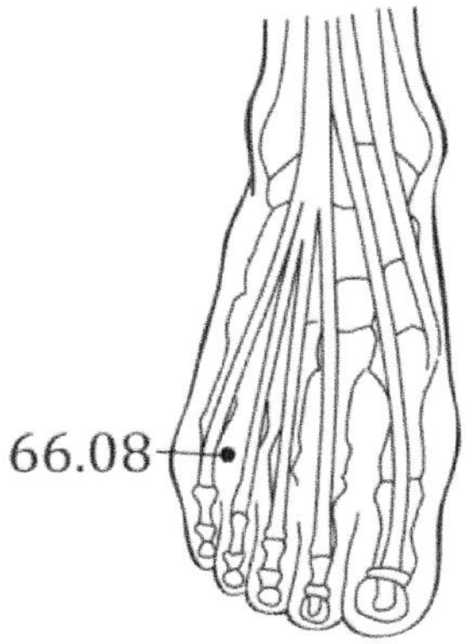

Liu Wan - Sixth Finish

Indications: Stops bleeding (including bleeding due to traumatic injury, incised wound, or injection), and migraine headaches.

Reaction areas: Lung, Kidney

Location: Between the 4th and 5th metatarsal bones, 0.5 cun proximal to the metatarsophalangeal joint. Points 66.08 and 66.09 are often used together.

66.09

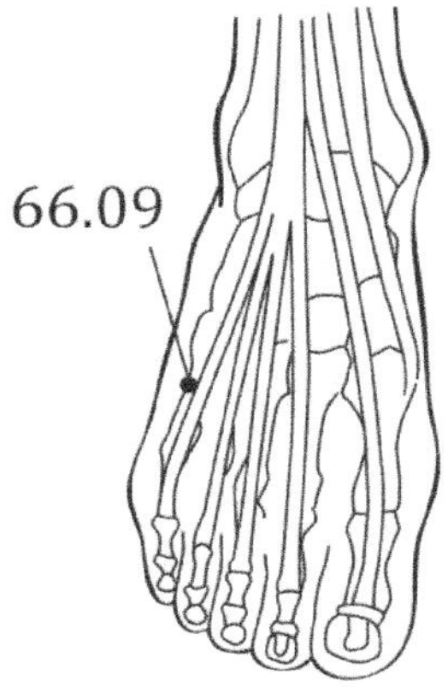

Shui Qu - Water Bend

Indications: Stops bleeding (including bleeding due to traumatic injury, incised wound, or injection), and migraine headaches. Lower back pain, edema, abdominal distension, generalized joint pain, neck pain caused by nerve problems, neuralgia of the neck, and uterine disorders.

Reaction areas: Lung, Kidney

Location: One cun proximal to 66.08. Located at the junction of the fourth and fifth toes, at the proximal metatarsal joint. Points 66.08 and 66.09 are usually used together.

66.10

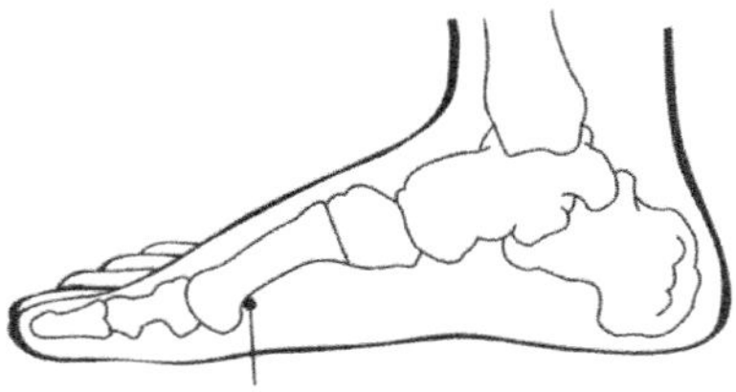

Huo Lian - Fire Lotus

Indications: Blurred vision and dizziness caused by hypertension, palpitations, and heart organ weakness.

Reaction areas: Heart, Kidney

Location: On the medial side of the first metatarsal bone, 1.5 cun posterior to the metatarsophalangeal joint. Located at Spleen 3.

66.11

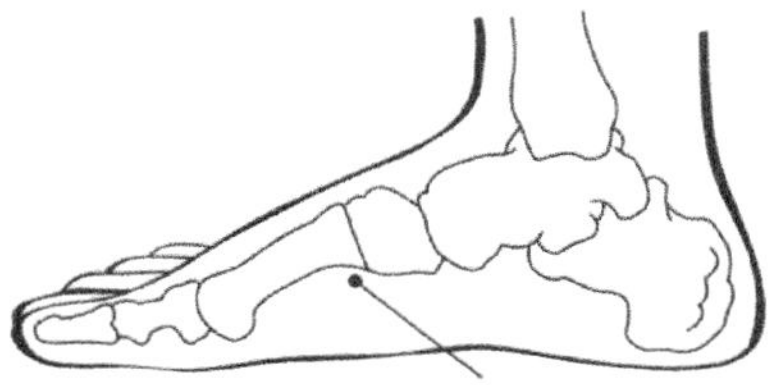

Huo Ju - Fire Chrysanthemum

Indications: Hand numbness, palpitations, dizziness, foot pain, hypertension, stiff neck, frontal headache, blurred vision, eyelid soreness, and eye disorders such as blurriness, difficulty focusing, floaters, and photophobia.

Reaction areas: Heart, Kidney

Location: One cun distal to 66.10. Insertion is .5 to 1 cun. Located at Spleen 4.

66.12

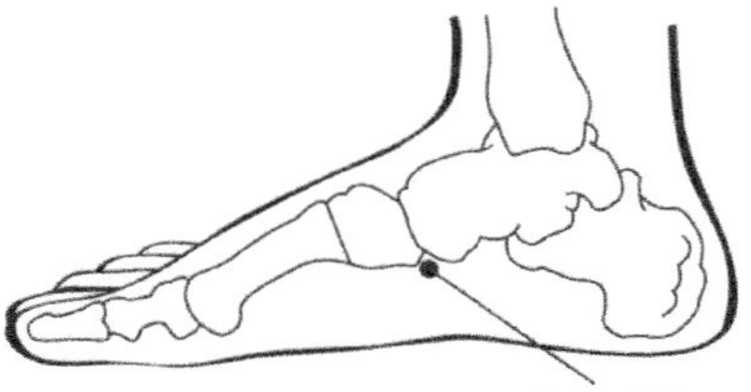

Huo San - Fire Scatter, Fire Powder

Indications: Headache, neck pain, dizziness, eye canthus pain, vision decline, lower back pain, blurred vision, conjunctivitis, kidney deficiency.

Reaction areas: Heart, Kidney, Six Fu- Bowels

Location: One cun posterior to 66.11

66.13

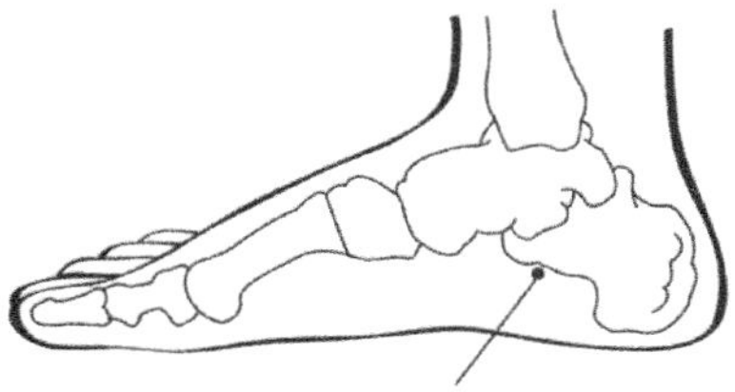

Shui Jing - Water Crystal

Indications: Uterine inflammation and tumors, distending sensation in the uterus, uterine tumor, abdominal distension, pelvic inflammatory disease, chocolate cysts.

Reaction area: Uterus

Location: Two cun inferior to the tip of the medial malleolus. The location is Kidney 6.

66.14

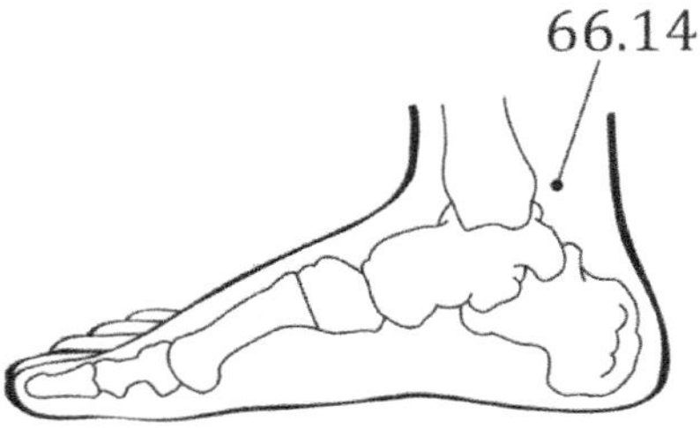

Shui Shang - Water Minister

Indications: Nephritis, lower back pain caused by kidney deficiency, spine pain, cataracts, febrile disease, pre-eclampsia, and limb edema. Postpartum fever.

Reaction areas: Brain, Kidneys

Location: Posterior to the medial malleolus, on the anterior border of the Achilles tendon, in the depression. Located at Kidney 3.

66.15

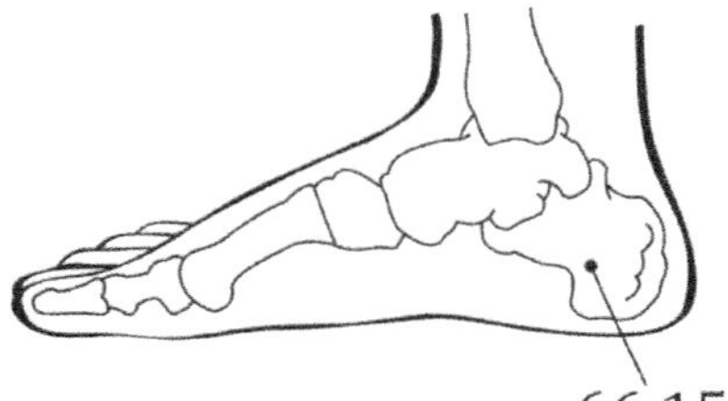

Shui Xian - Water Immortal

Indications: The same as 66.14. (Nephritis, lower back pain caused by kidney deficiency, spine pain, cataracts, febrile disease, pre-eclampsia, and edema.)

Reaction areas: Brain, Kidneys

Location: Two cun posterior to the medial malleolus, in the depression at the anterior border of the Achilles tendon. This is 2 cun below Kidney 3.

77.01, 77.02, 77.03, 77.04

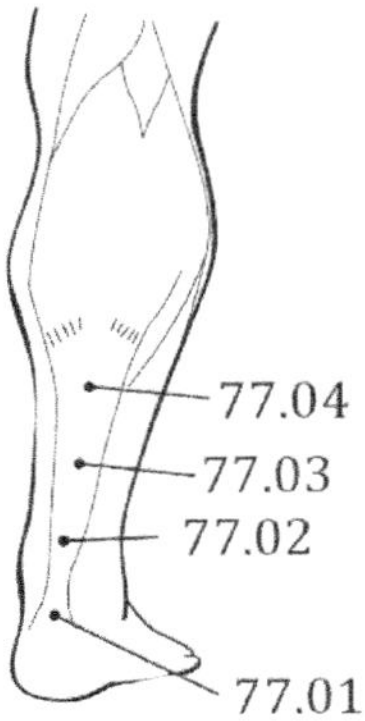

77.01, Zheng Jin, Upright Tendon
77.02, Zheng Zong, Upright Ancestor
77.03, Zheng Shi, Upright Master
77.04, Bo Qiu, Catching Ball

Straight Spine Dao Ma

Indications: Neck pain or sprain, spinal pain, neck rigidity, lower back pain, vertebral pain due to sprain, lumbar vertebral pain, neck pain and rigidity and cranial enlargement and hydrocephalus. Pain in the shoulder and back, lower back pain, and sciatica

Reaction areas: Brain, Spine

77.01, 77.02, 77.03, 77.04

Location: In the center of the calcaneus tendon, 3.5 cun superior to the heel. Perpendicular insertion. You must tap the posterior side of the tibia. Insert the needle through the Achilles tendon. 77.01 is 3.5 cun superior to the sole of the foot, on the Achilles tendon. At the level of the tip of the lateral malleolus and BL 60. Other authors locate this point on a range of 2.5 to 4.5 cun from the sole of the foot.

77.02 is two cun superior to 77.01. 77.03 is two cun superior to 77.02. 77.04 is two and a half cun superior to 77.03.

77.05, 77.06, 77.07

Three Weights Dao Ma

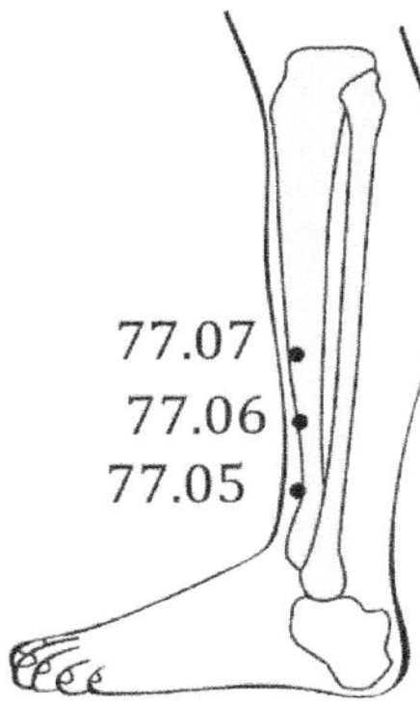

77.05, Yi Zhong, First Weight
77.06, Er Zhong, Second Weight
77.07, San Zhong, Third Weight

Indications: Hyperthyroidism, tonsillitis, deviation of the eye and mouth, migraine headaches, mastitis, fibrocystic breast disease, breast tumors, meningitis, liver disease, splenomegaly, lateral side rib pain, abnormally bulging eyes, lumps, Bell's palsy, and brain tumors.

Reaction areas: Heart, Lung, Spleen

77.05, 77.06, 77.07

Three Weights Dao Ma

Location:

77.05 is 3 cun proximal to the lateral malleolus, and 1 cun anterior to the fibula

77.06 is 2 cun proximal to 77.05

77.07 is 2 cun proximal to 77.06

Insertion is 1 to 2 cun.

77.08

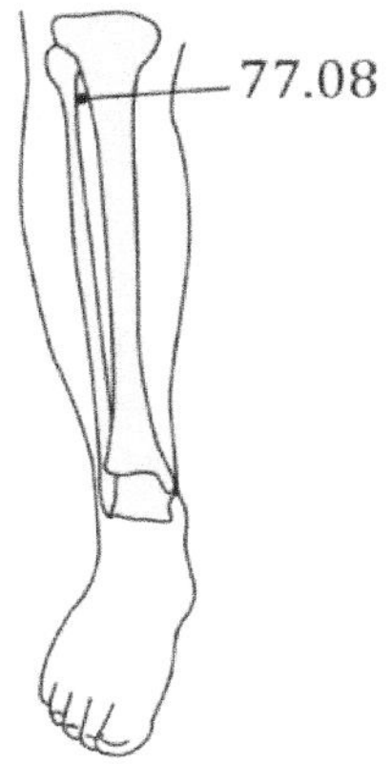

Si Hua Shang - Four Flowers Upper

Indications: Asthma, toothache, dizziness, palpitations, coronary artery disease, vomiting, and sudden turmoil.

Reaction areas: Lung, Heart

Location: Three cun inferior to ST 35 on the lateral side of the tibia. Insertion is 2 to 3.5 cun.

77.09

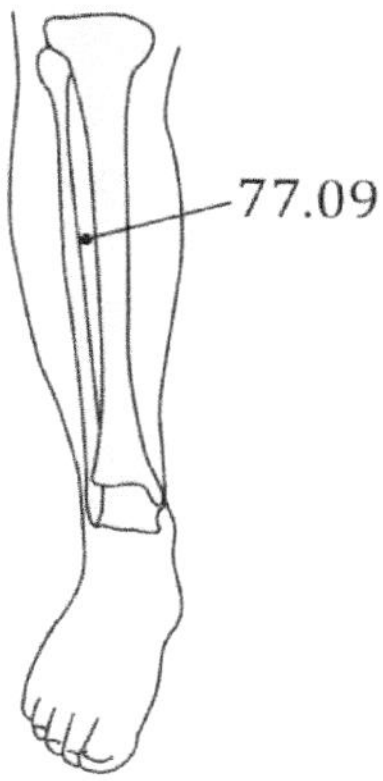

Si Hua Zhong - Four Flowers Middle

Indications: Asthma, heart pain, sensation of chest suffocation or discomfort, eye problems, stomach pain, and swollen bones, heart organ paralysis.

Reaction areas: Heart, Lung.

Location: 4.5 cun inferior to 77.08. Insertion is 2 to 3 cun.

77.10

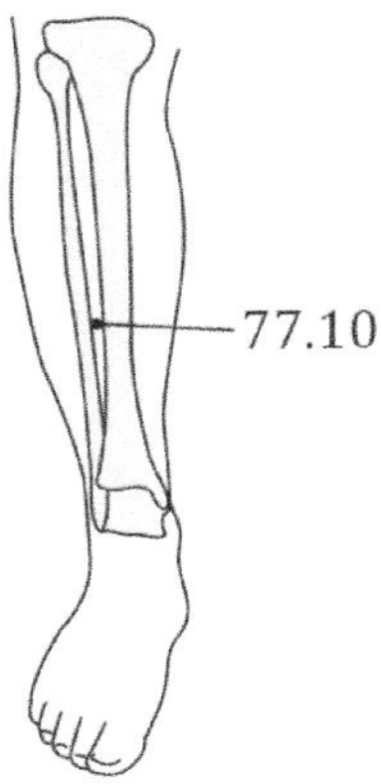

Si Hua Fu - Four Flowers Append

Indications: Asthma, carditis, heart pain, sensation of chest suffocation, acute stomach pain, eye problem.

Reaction area: Heart and lung

Location: 2.5 cun inferior to 77.09.

77.11

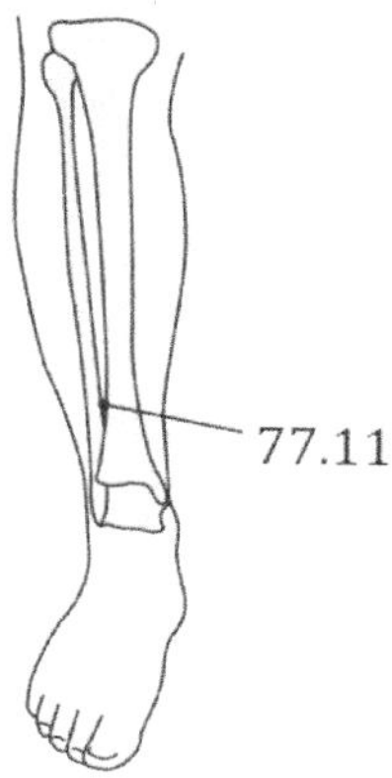

Si Hua Xia - Four Flowers Lower

Indications: Edema, enteritis, abdominal distention, and teeth grinding.

Location: 2.5 cun below 77.10.

77.12

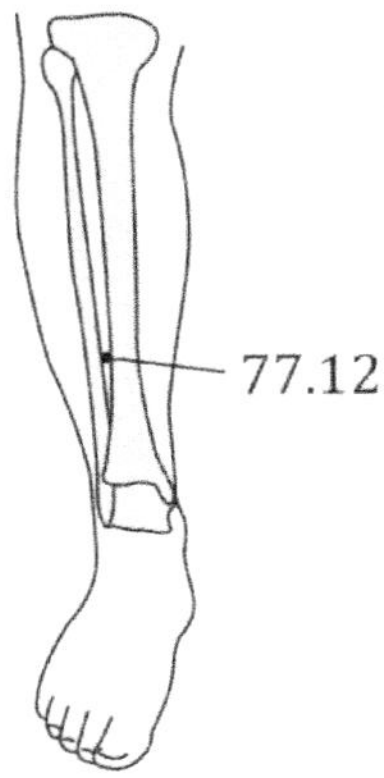

Fu Chang - Bowel Intestine

Indications: Teeth grinding, bone spurs (touch the bone), enteritis, abdominal distension, stomach pain, edema.

Location: 1.5 cun above 77.11.

77.13

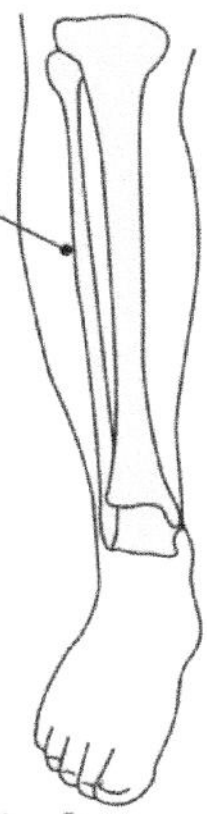

Si Hua Li - Inner Four Flowers

Indications: Heart diseases, palpitations, gastritis, vomiting, knee osteoarthritis, coronary artery disease.

Location: On the inner border of the tibia bone, 1.2 cun medial to 77.09. Insertion is 1.5 to 2 cun.

77.14

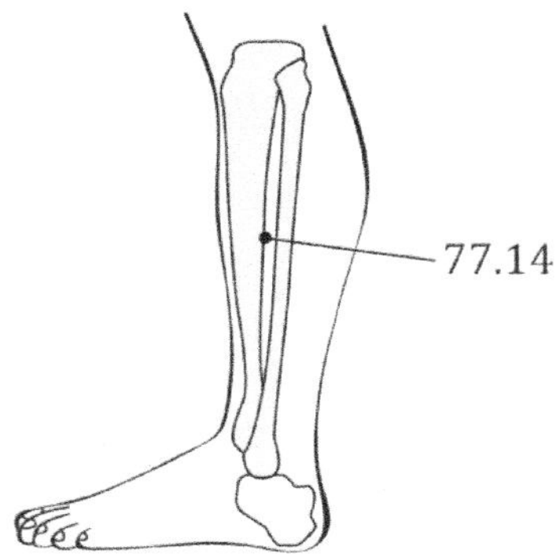

Si Hua Wai - Lateral Four Flowers

Indications: Toothache, migraine headache (can be bled), facial paralysis, Bell's palsy, intercostal neuralgia, ear pain, tennis elbow, shoulder and arm pain, sciatica, instep pain, hypertension, acute inflammation of the intestines.

Location: 1.5 cun lateral to 77.09. Insertion 1 to 1.5 cun.

77.15, 77.16

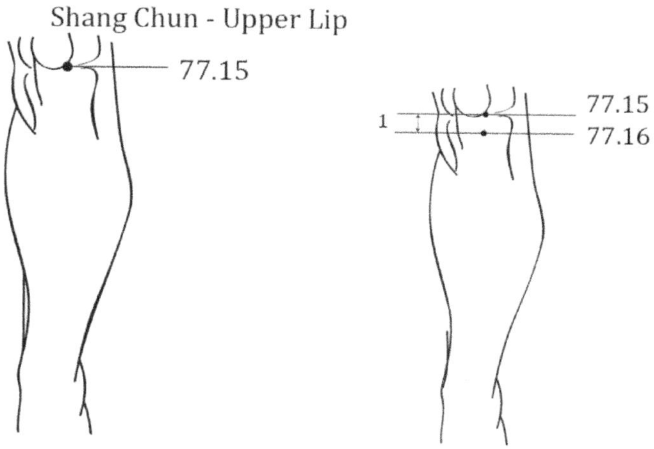

77.15, Shang Chun, Upper Lip

Indications: Lip pain, mouth ulcerations, vitiligo around the mouth or genitals.

Location: Lower lateral ridge of the patella. The point can be bled until dark red blood appears.

77.16, Xia Chun, Lower Lip

Indications: Lip pain, vitiligo around the mouth or genitals.

Location: One cun below the lower lateral ridge of the patella. The point can be bled.

77.17

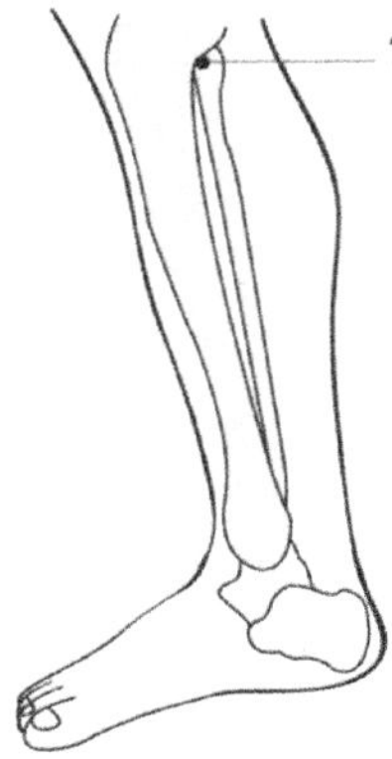

Tian Huang - Heavenly Emperor

Indications: This point is Spleen 9. Rheumatoid arthritis, hypertension, diabetes, proteinuria, nephritis, insomnia, acid reflux, stomach acid disorders, arm pain.

Reaction areas: Kidney and Heart

Location: On the medial condyle of the tibia bone, 2.5 cun below the knee joint.

77.18

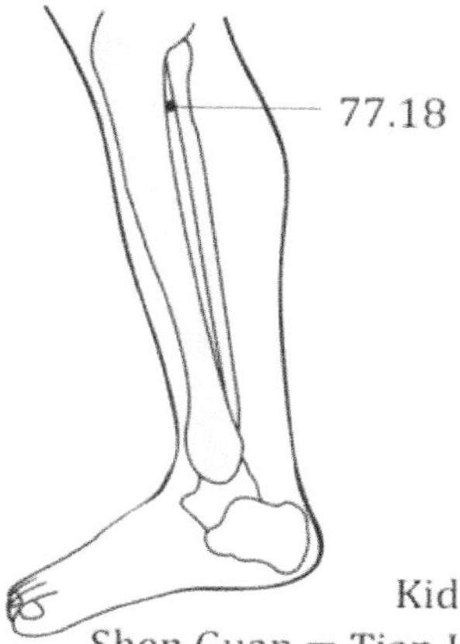

Kidney Gate
Shen Guan = Tian Huang Fu

Indications: Edema, kidney disease, diabetes mellitus, strangury, premature ejaculation, impotence, incontinence, seminal emission, nocturnal emission, hematuria, uterine tumors, nephritis, edema of the limbs, proteinuria, irregular menstruation, and lower back pain due to kidney deficiency. Trigeminal neuralgia, fatigue and weakness, general digestive problems, gynecological disorders, and male genital problems such as prostate issues. Kidney tonic point.

Reaction area: Kidney

Location: This point is 1.5 cun distal to SP 9. Insertion is 1-2 cun.

77.19

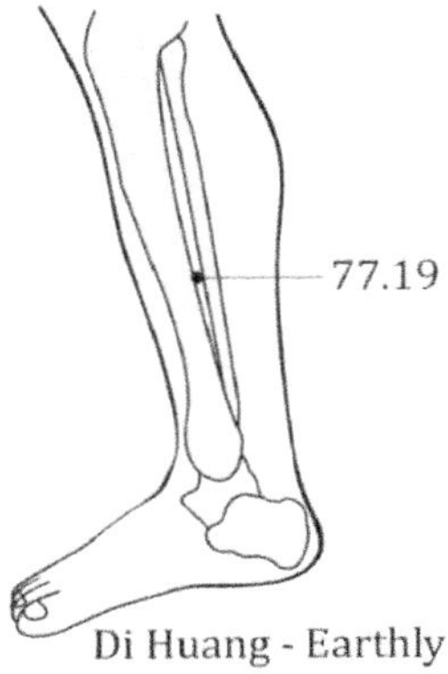

Di Huang - Earthly Emperor

Indications: Edema, kidney disease, diabetes mellitus, strangury, premature ejaculation, impotence, seminal emission, nocturnal emission, hematuria, uterine tumors, nephritis, edema of the limbs, proteinuria, tumors of the uterus, irregular menstruation, lower back pain due to kidney deficiency.

Reaction area: Kidney

Location: Located 7 cun proximal to the tip of the medial malleolus, on the SP channel.

77.20

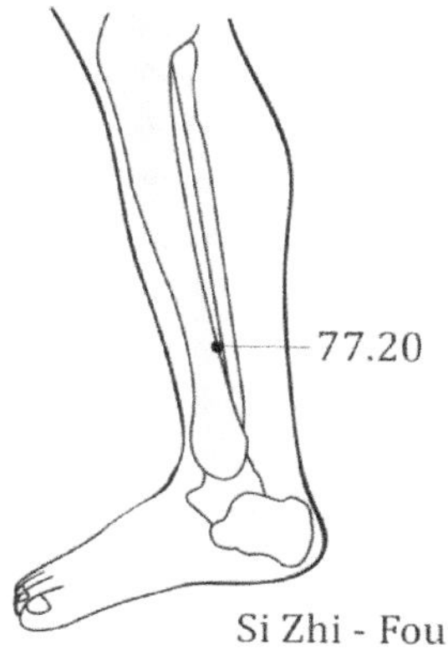

Si Zhi - Four Limbs

Indications: Neck pain, arm pain, diabetes, hand pain, and foot pain.

Location: 4 cun superior to the lateral malleolus, on the medial side of the tibia.

77.21

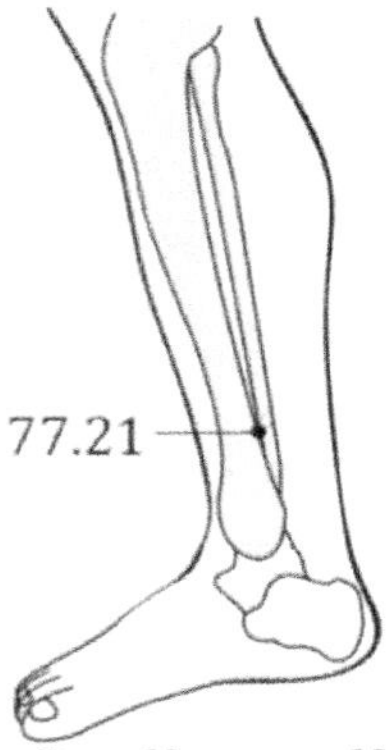

Ren Huang - Human Emperor

Indications: Edema, kidney disease, diabetes mellitus, strangury, premature ejaculation, impotence, seminal emission, nocturnal emission, hematuria, uterine tumors, nephritis, proteinuria, irregular menstruation, and lower back pain due to deficiency of the kidneys. Trigeminal neuralgia, fatigue and weakness, general digestive and gynecological disorders. This point is very close to SP 6, and thus it has many of the same indications of that point.

Reaction area: Kidney

Location: Located three cun above the tip of the medial malleolus, on the SP channel. Located at SP 6.

77.22, 77.23

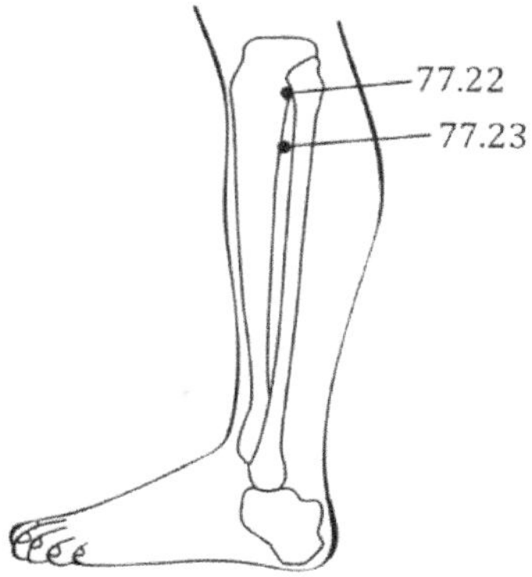

77.22, Ce San Li, Beside Three Miles
77.23, Ce Xia San Li, Distal to Beside Three Miles

Indications: Toothache, facial paralysis, headache, sinusitis, trigeminal neuralgia, Bell's palsy, carpal tunnel, teeth and mouth problems, heel pain, and facial tics.

Reaction area: Teeth, Lung

Location: Point 77.22 is 1.5 cun lateral to ST 36. Point 77.23 is 2 cun distal to 77.22, on the anterior border of the fibula.

77.24

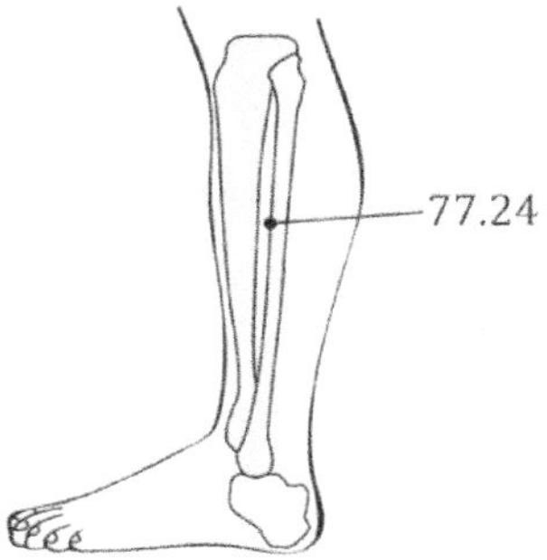

Zu Qian Jin - Leg 1000 Gold

Indications: Acute intestinal inflammation, throat abscesses, laryngitis, tonsillitis, thyroiditis, back pain, shoulder pain, fish bone stuck in throat, plum pit Qi

Reaction areas: Lung, Kidney and Thyroid

Location: .5 cun lateral and 2 cun inferior to 77.23. Insertion is 1 to 2 cun.

77.25

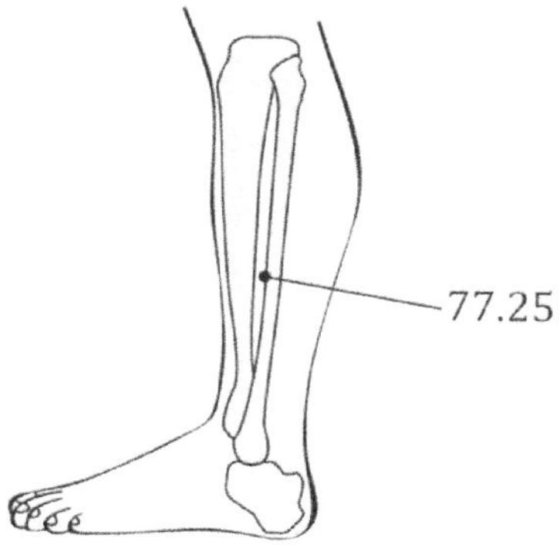

Zu Wu Jin - Leg Five Gold

Indications: Acute intestinal inflammation, fish bone stuck in the throat, shoulder pain, throat abscess, pharyngitis, thyroid enlargement.

Reaction areas: Lung, Kidney, and Thryoid

Location: 2 cun inferior to 77.24.

77.26

Qi Hu - Seven Tigers

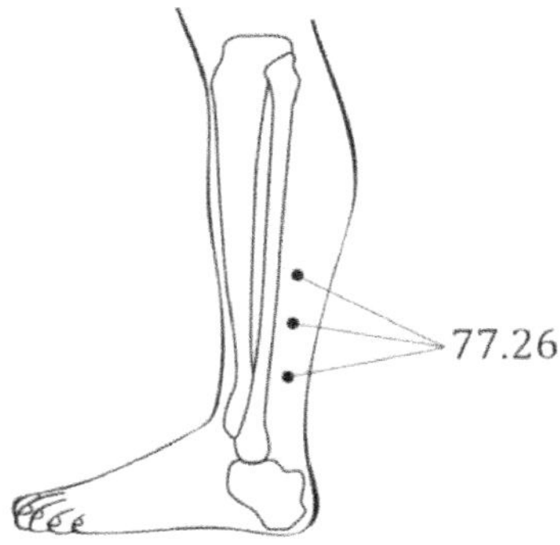

Indications: Sternum pain, clavicle pain, rib pain, and pleurisy.

Reaction areas: Chest, Thoracic cage

Location: Located 1.5 cun posterior to the lateral malleolus, on the BL channel. The first point is 2 cun above the tip of the lateral malleolus, the second point is 4 cun above the tip, and the third is 6 cun above the tip. Located behind the posterior border of the fibula.

77.27

Wai San Guan - Outer Three Gates

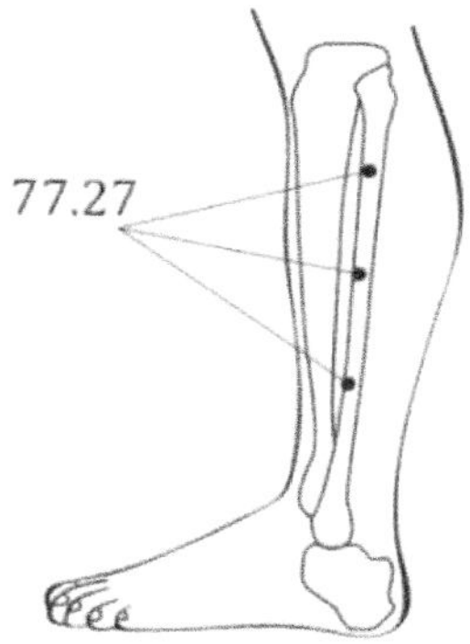

Three Lateral Passes Dao Ma

Indications: Tonsillitis, mumps, laryngitis, abscesses, tumors, and pain in the shoulder and arm.

Reaction area: Lung

Location: This is a three point unit, located on the line that connects the head of the fibula and the lateral malleolus. The points are located at the ¼, ½, and ¾ units. Tap the tibia for the best results. Insertion is 1 to 1.5 cun.

77.28

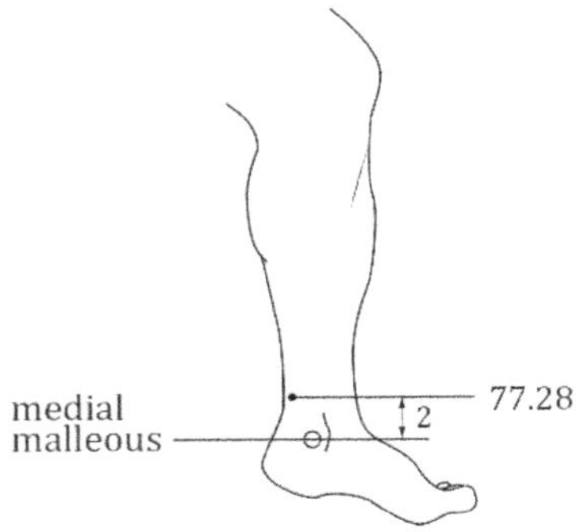

77.28, Guang Ming, Bright Eye

Indications: Kidney weakness, eye diseases such as astigmatism, cataracts, double vision, glaucoma, drooping eyelids, diabetic retinopathy, peripheral neuropathy.

Location: One cun posterior to and 2 cun superior to the medial malleolus. Insertion .5 to 1 cun deep. This point overlaps Kidney 7.

88.01, 88.02, 88.03

Three Penetrations Dao Ma

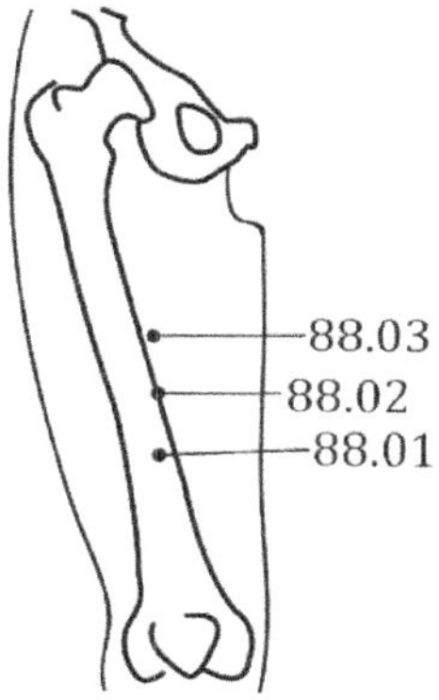

88.01, Tong Guan, Penetrating Gate
88.02, Tong Shan, Penetrating Mountain
88.03, Tong Tian, Penetrating Heaven

Three Penetrations Dao Ma

Indications: Heart disease, pericardium pain, pain on both sides of the heart, dizziness, vertigo, gastric disease, palpitations, rheumatic heart disease, limb pain, acute pericarditis, cerebral ischemia, rheumatic fever, and nausea and vomiting in pregnancy.

Reaction area: Heart

88.01, 88.02, 88.03

Three Penetrations Dao Ma

Locations:

88.01 is located on the anterior midline of the femur, 5 cun superior to the knee crease.

88.02 is located 2 cun more proximal, or a total of 7 cun proximal from the knee crease.

88.03 is located 2 cun more proximal or a total of 9 cun proximal from the knee crease.

88.04, 88.05, 88.06

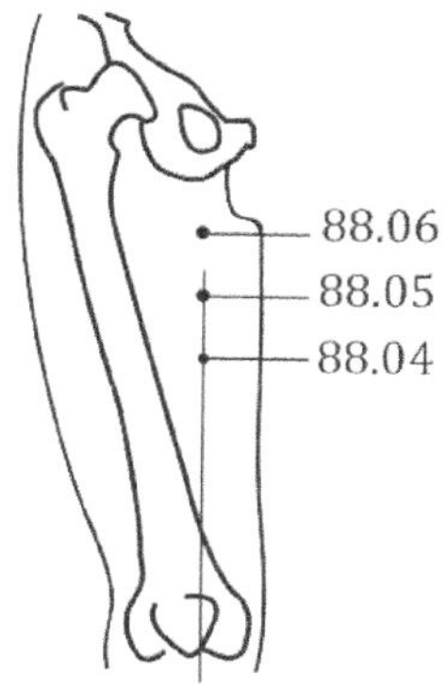

88.04, Jie Mei Yi, Sister One

Indications: Uterine tumors, irregular menses, vaginal itching, stomach hemorrhage, intestinal pain, uterine inflammation.

Location: One cun medial to and 1 cun superior to 88.02.

88.05, Jie Mei Er, Sister Two

Indications: Uterine tumors, irregular menses, vaginal itching, stomach hemorrhage, intestinal pain, uterine inflammation.

Location: 2.5 cun above 88.04

88.04, 88.05, 88.06

88.06, Jie Mei San, Sister Three

Indications: Uterine tumors, irregular menses, vaginal itching, stomach hemorrhage, intestinal pain, uterine inflammation.

Location: 2.5 cun above 88.05

88.07, 88.08

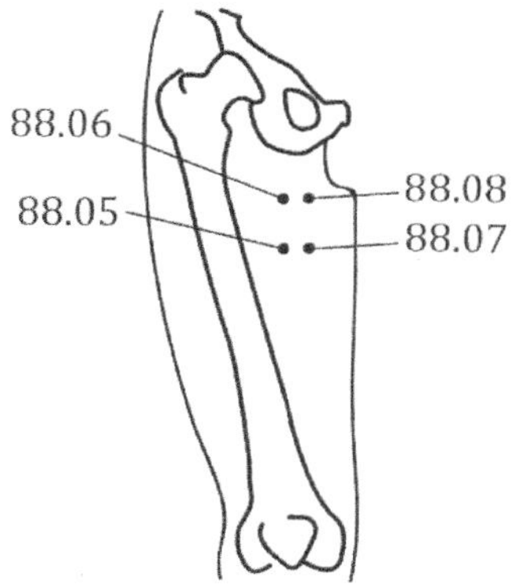

88.07, Gan Mao Yi, Common Cold One

Indications: High fever, severe common cold, headache during cold or flu.

Location: One cun medial to 88.05

88.08, Gan Mao Er, Common Cold Two

Indications: High fever, severe common cold, headache during cold or flu

Location: One cun medial to 88.06

88.09, 88.10, 88.11

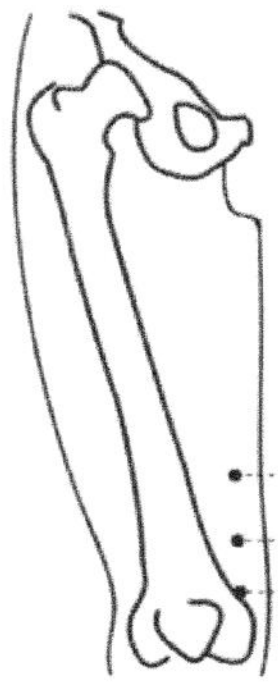

88.09, Tong Shen, Penetrating Kidney

Indications for 88.09, 88.10, and 88.11 include Impotence, premature ejaculation, painful urination, nephritis, lower back pain, uterine pain, red or white vaginal discharge, and diabetes.

Location: On the medial side, superior border of the patella.

Reaction area: Kidney

88.10, Tong Wei, Penetrating Stomach
Location: 2 cun superior to 88.09

88.11, Tong Bei, Penetrating Back
Location: 4 cun superior to 88.09

88.12, 88.13, 88.14

Three Upper Yellow Dao Ma

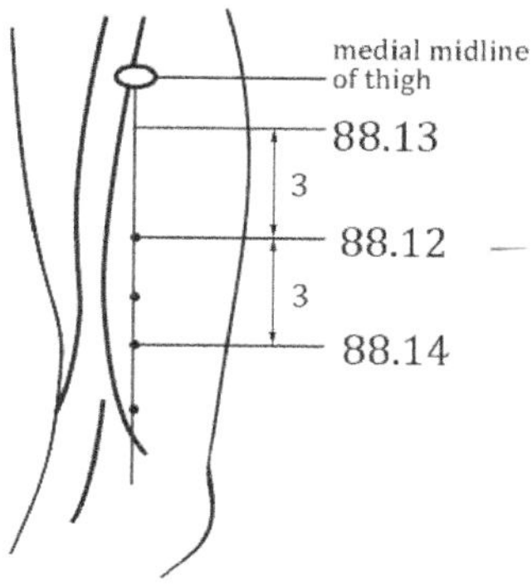

88.12, Ming Huang, Bright Yellow
88.13, Tian Huang, Heavenly Yellow
88.14, Qi Huang, Other Yellow

Three Upper Yellow Dao Ma

Indications: Liver cirrhosis, hepatitis, body swelling, fatigue, back pain, chorea (which is involuntary jerky movements, as seen in Parkinson's disease), leukemia, multiple sclerosis (especially with double vision). Liver cirrhosis, hepatitis, enlargement of bones, spinal meningitis, fatigue due to hypofunction of the Liver, soreness of the lower back, blurred vision, eye pain, liver pain, indigestion.

88.12, 88.13, 88.14

Reaction areas: Kidney (superficial depth). Liver (middle depth), Heart (deep level).

Location: In the center of the medial aspect of the thigh.

88.12 is located on the midpoint of the inner thigh on the LV channel.
88.13 is located 3 cun proximal to 88.12 on the LV channel.
88.14 is located 3 cun distal to 88.12 on the LV channel.

Insertion is 1.5 to 2.5 cun.

88.15

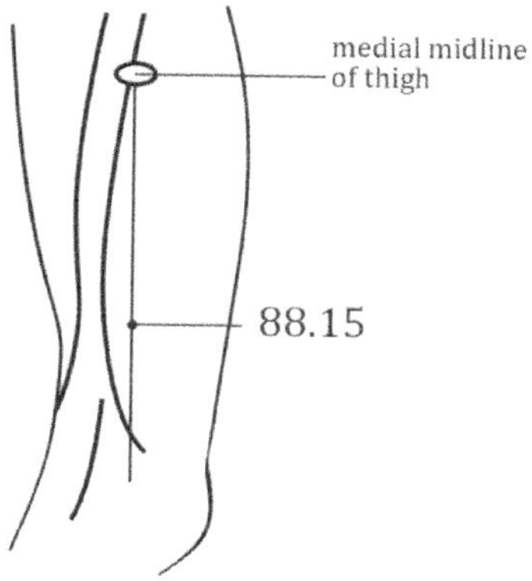

Huo Zhi - Fire Branch

88.15, Huo Zhi, Fire Branch

Indications: Jaundice and dizziness due to liver patterns, gallstones, gallbladder inflammation, back pain, blurred vision.

Location: 1.5 cun above 88.14. Insertion is 1.5 to 2 cun.

88.16

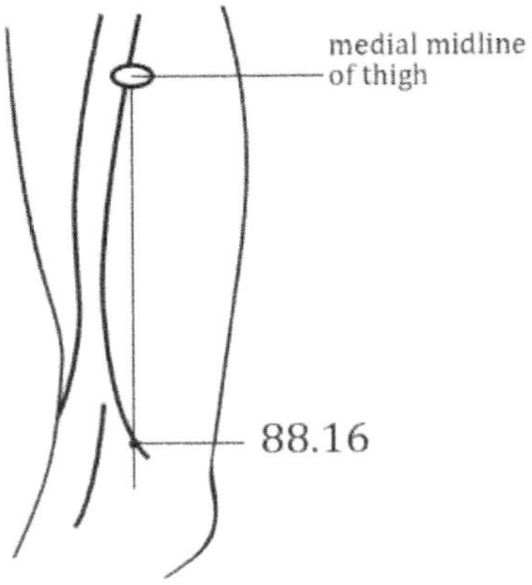

Huo Quan - Fire Complete

88.16, Huo Quan, Fire Complete

Indications the same as 88.15. Jaundice and dizziness due to liver patterns, gallstones, back pain, blurred vision.

Location: 1.5 cun below 88.14

88.17, 88.18, 88.19

Three Upper Horses Dao Ma, or Si Ma Points

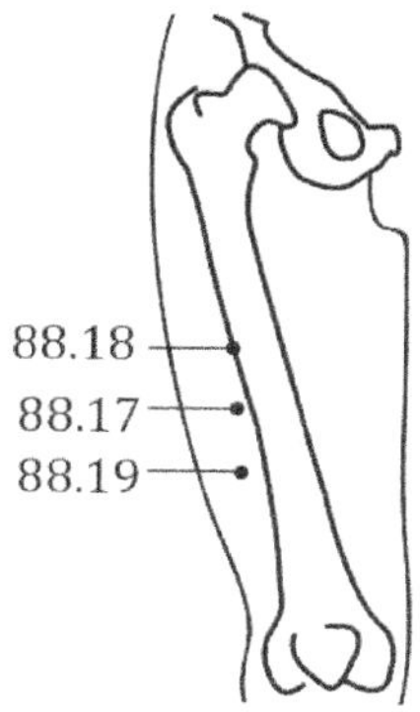

88.17, Si Ma Zhong, Rapid Horses Center
88.18, Si Ma Shang, Rapid Horses Upper
88.19, Si Ma Xia, Rapid Horses Lower
Three Upper Horses or Si Ma Points Dao Ma

Indications: Hypochondriac pain, back pain, sciatica and lower back pain due to hypofunction of the lungs, pneumonia, tuberculosis, chest and back pain due to injury, pleurisy, rhinitis, deafness, tinnitus, otitis, dermatitis, facial paralysis, congested eyes, asthma, breast pain, hemiplegia, psoriasis, dermatosis, and strain of the lower limbs. Lateral side rib pain, sciatica, chest pain, pulmonary tuberculosis, conjunctivitis, breast pain, rhinitis, and dermatological disorders.

88.17, 88.18, 88.19

Reaction areas: Liver, Lung

Location: Three cun anterior to the spot touched by the middle fingertip when one is standing with his hands at his sides.

88.20, 88.21, 88.22

Three Springs Dao Ma

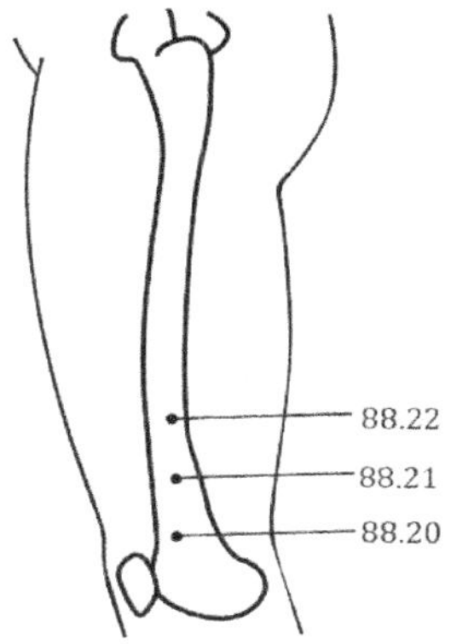

88.20, Xia Quan, Lower Spring
88.21, Zhong Quan, Center Spring
88.22, Shang Quan, Upper Spring

Indications: Facial paralysis, facial tics, deviation of the eyes and mouth, tinnitus, poor hearing, and Bell's palsy.

Reaction areas: Face, Lung

Location: Perpendicular insertion, through the IT band. Touch the bone on insertion.

88.20, 88.21, 88.22

88.20 Two and a half cun superior to the knee joint, on the medial line of the lateral thigh.
88.21 Two cun superior to 88.20.
88.22 Two cun superior to 88.21.

88.23, 88.24

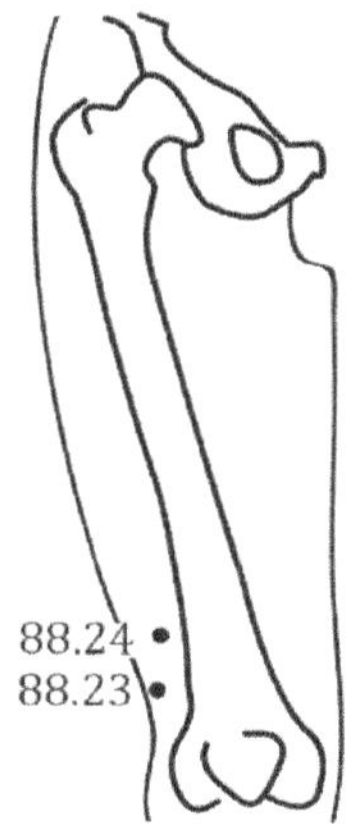

88.23, Jin Zian Xia, Gold Front Lower

Indications: Lung and liver deficiency, epilepsy, headache, indigestion, skin allergies.

Location: One cun superior to the outer border of the patella. Insertion is .3 to .5 cun.

88.24, Jin Qian Shang, Gold Front Upper

Indications: Lung and liver deficiency, epilepsy, headache, indigestion, skin allergies.

Location: 1.5 cun superior to 88.23. Insertion is .5 to 1 cun.

88.25

Zhong Jiu Li - Center Nine Miles

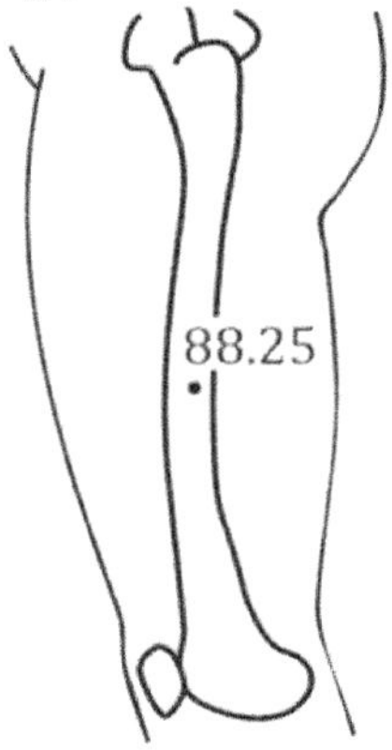

Indications: Back pain, lower back pain, lumbar vertebral pain, hemiplegia, facial paralysis, neck pain, and dizziness, distending feeling in the eyes, numbness of the hand and arm and leg. Lateral thigh pain, migraine headaches, cervical spondylosis, facial pain, tinnitus, leg or knee pain, bone spurs, and lack of strength in the nerves.

Reaction areas: All four limbs, Lung

Location: This point is located in the same location as the TCM point GB 31. It is in the middle of the femur. For best results insert to touch the bone.

88.26

Shang Jiu Li - Upper Nine Miles

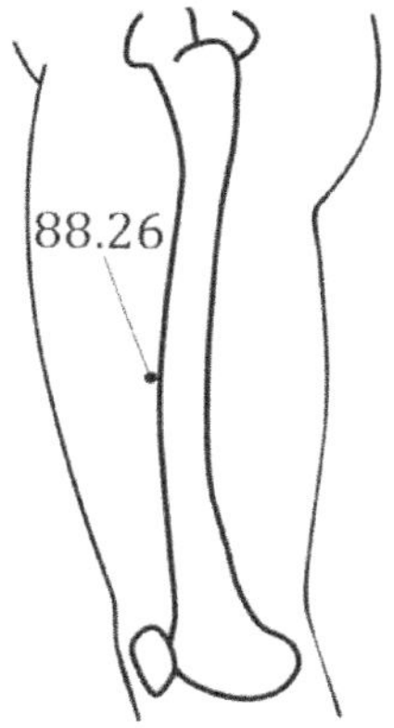

Indications: Arm pain due to heart channel stagnation, eye pain, and abdominal pain due to kidney weakness.

Location: 1.5 cun anterior to 88.25.

88.27

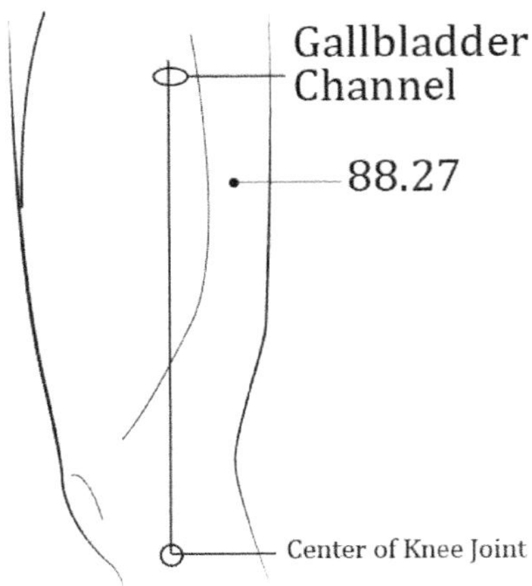

Xia Jiu Li - Lower Nine Miles

Indications: Back pain, leg pain, and thigh pain.

Location: 1.5 cun posterior to 88.25.

88.28

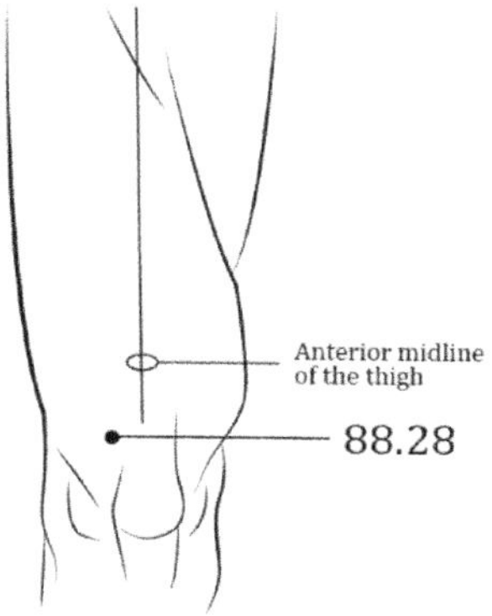

Jie - Release Point

Indications: Pain from trauma, swelling around acupuncture treatment site, pain from injection, extreme fatigue, generalized pain.

Location: One third of a cun proximal to 1 cun superior to the outer edge of the patella.

88.29

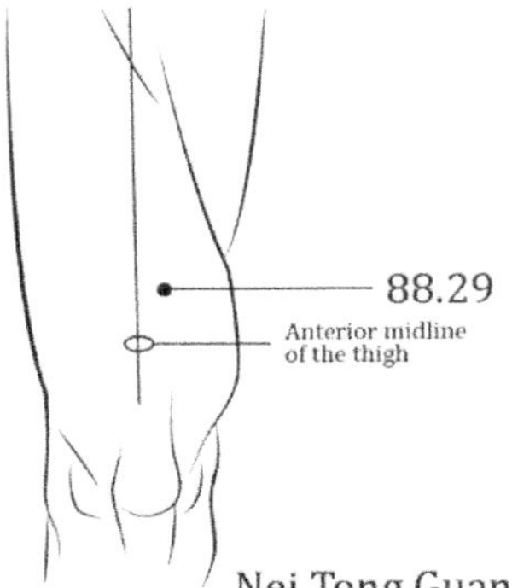

Nei Tong Guan -
Inner Penetrating Gate

Indications: Limb weakness, hemiplegia, palpitations, wind stroke, heart hypofunction, lower back pain, inability to raise the hands, transient ischemic attacks, weak limbs, aphasia due to stroke.

Location: .5 cun medial to 88.01.

88.30

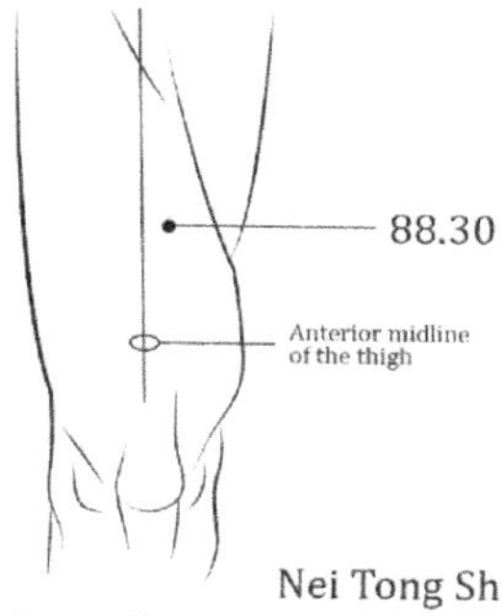

Nei Tong Shen
Inner Penetrating Mountain

Indications: Limb weakness, hemiplegia, palpitations, wind stroke, heart hypofunction, lower back pain, inability to raise the hands, transient ischemic attacks, weak limbs, aphasia due to stroke.

Location: .5 cun medial to 88.02.

88.31

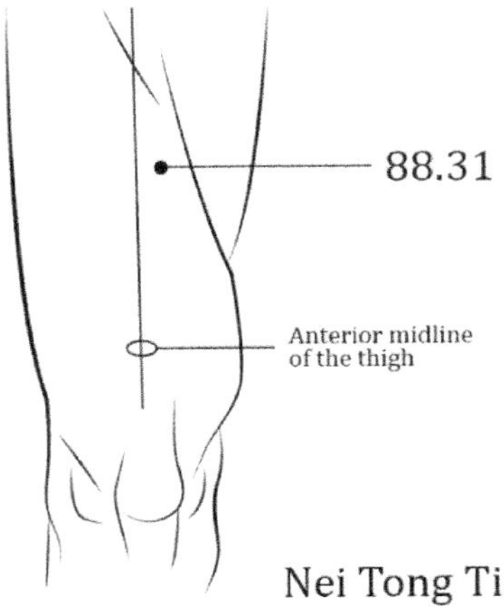

Nei Tong Tian
Inner Penetrating Heaven

Indications: Limb weakness, hemiplegia, palpitations, wind stroke, heart hypofunction, lower back pain, inability to raise the hands, transient ischemic attacks, weak limbs, aphasia due to stroke.

Location: .5 cun medial to 88.03.

88.32

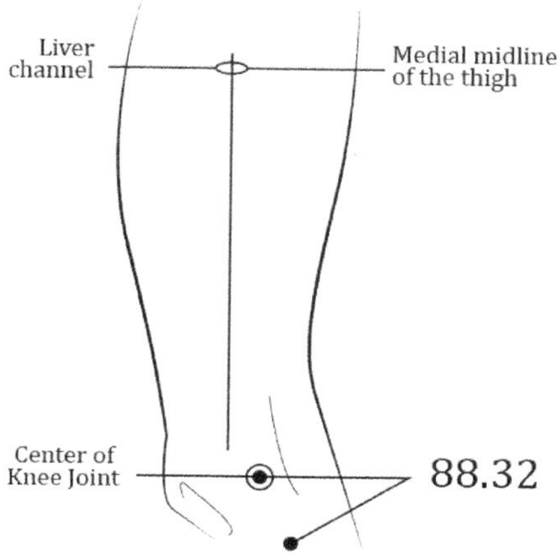

Shi Yin - Sound of Voice

Indications: Tonsillitis, inability to produce voiced sound (aphonia), hoarse voice, thyroiditis, parathyroiditis, swollen throat. (A common cause of aphonia is damage to the laryngeal nerve, which supplies most of the muscles in the larynx. This damage can be caused by surgery, or thyroidectomy.)

Location: A two point unit. The first point is in the center of the medial patella, and the second point is inferior to that. Insertion is 2 cun.

99.01 to 99.08

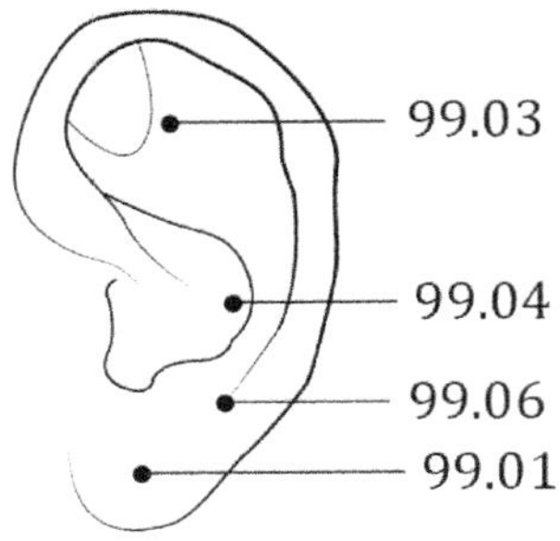

99.01
Er Huan
Ear Ring
Intoxication from alcohol and vomiting.
In the center of the ear lobe.

99.03
Hou Er
Fire Ear
Heart failure, knee, and limb pain.
In the middle of the outer border of the antihelix.

99.04
Tu Er
Earth Ear
Neurasthenia, polycythemia, high fever, and diabetes.
In the center of the cavity of the concha.

99.06
Shui Er
Water Ear

Kidney deficiency, pain on both sides of the lower back, and abdominal distension.

At the lower end of the outer border of antihelix.

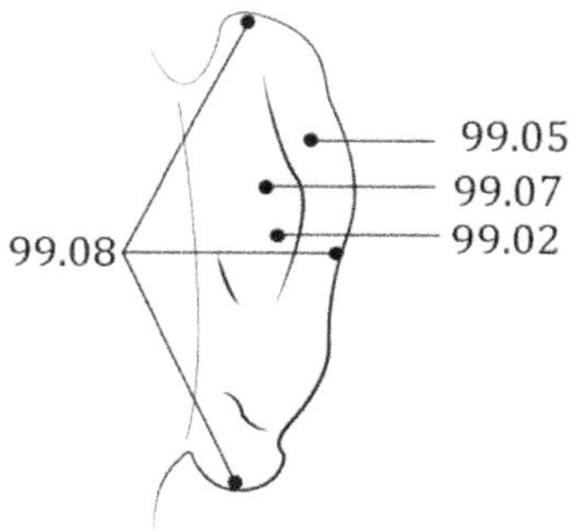

99.02
Mu Er
Wood Ear

Liver pain, hepatomegaly, hepatocirrhosis, and fatigue due to deficiency in the Liver, and chronic strangury.

Longitudinally, 0.3 cun below the middle transverse branch of the dorsal auricular artery of the posterior side of the ear.

99.01 to 99.08

99.05
Jin Er
Wood Ear

Sciatica due to hypofunction of the Lung, lumbar vertebra bending and allergic common cold.

One third of a cun superior to Shui Er (99.06).

99.07
Er Bei
Back of Ear

Pharyngitis and tonsillitis.

About 0.33 cun above Mu Er (99.03).

Bleed the point with a three-edged needle.

99.08
Er San
Ear Three

Cholera, migraine, common cold, and tonsillitis.

On the outer border of the helix of the ear.

Bleed the points with a three-edged needle.

1010.01

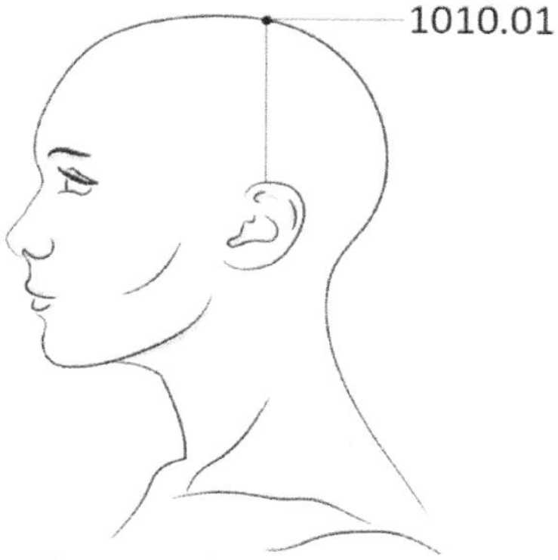

Zheng Hui - Upright Meeting

Indications: Hemiplegia, fatigue, tremors, infantile convulsions, eye and mouth deviation (from stroke), aphasia due to stroke, dysfunction of nervous system, stroke sequellae, cerebral palsy.

Reaction areas: Brain, Cerebral nerve

Location: Located at Du 20. Perpendicular insertion. Insertion is .1 to .3 cun.

1010.02, 1010.03, 1010.04

Zhou Yuan - Prefecture Round

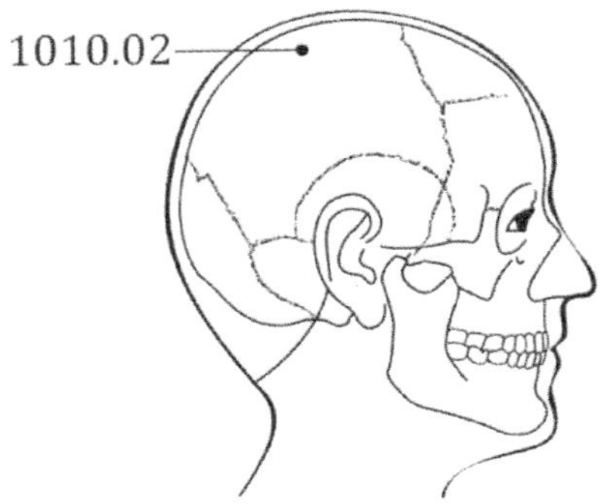

Zhou Kun - Prefecture Elder Brother

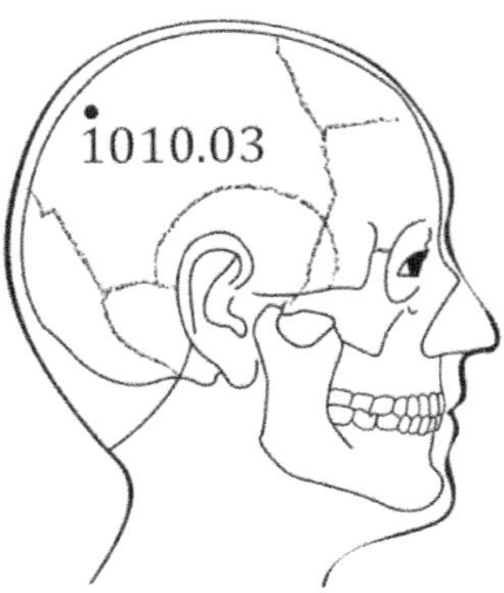

1010.02, 1010.03, 1010.04

Zhou Lun - Prefecture Mountain

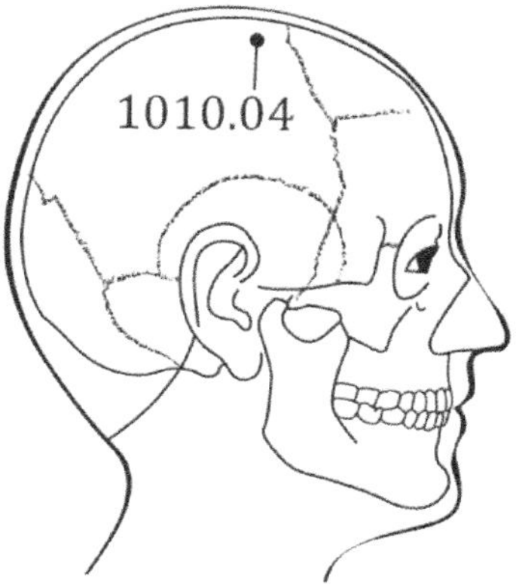

1010.02

Indications: Asthma, lower back pain, sciatica, shortness of breath.

Reaction area: Lung

Location: 1.5 cun lateral to 1010.01

1010.03

Indications: Asthma, lower back pain, sciatica, shortness of breath. Hemiplegia, limb weakness.

Location: 1.5 cun posterior to 1010.02

1010.02, 1010.03, 1010.04

1010.04

Indications: Asthma, lower back pain, sciatica, shortness of breath. Hemiplegia, limb weakness, brain tumor.

Reaction area: Lung

Location: 1.5 cun anterior to 1010.02.

1010.05

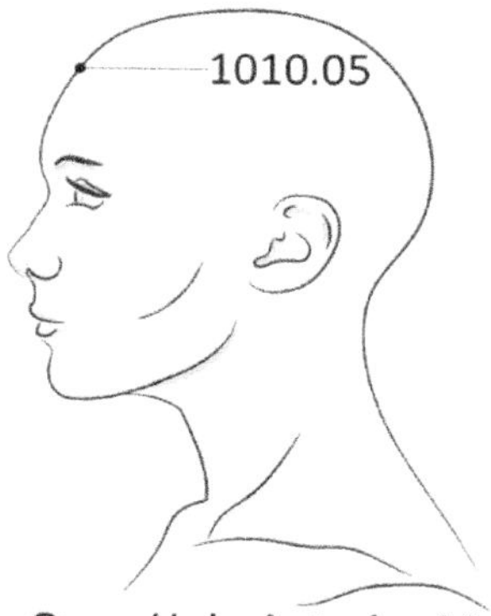

Quan Hui - Anterior Meeting

Indications: Dizziness, blurred vision, distending feeling of the head, and neurasthenia, which is physical and mental exhaustion.

Reaction area: Brain

Location: One and a half cun anterior to 1010.01. Insertion is .1 to .3 cun.

1010.06

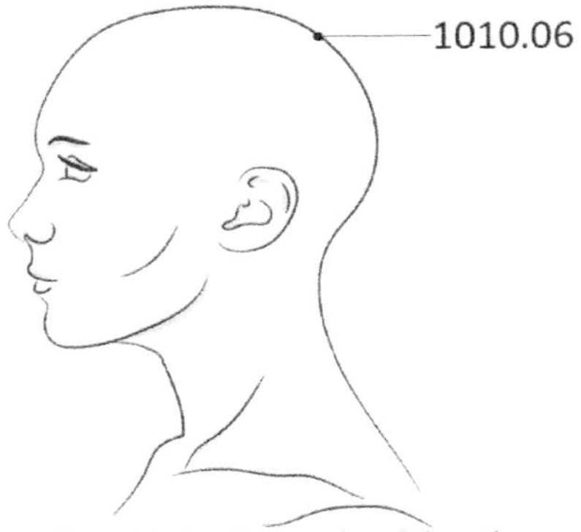

Hou Hui - Posterior Meeting

Indications: Bone tuberculosis, dizziness, headaches, spinal pain, and stroke.

Reaction areas: Brain, Spine

Location: Located 1.6 cun posterior to 1010.01. Perpendicular insertion. Insertion is .1 to .3 cun.

1010.07

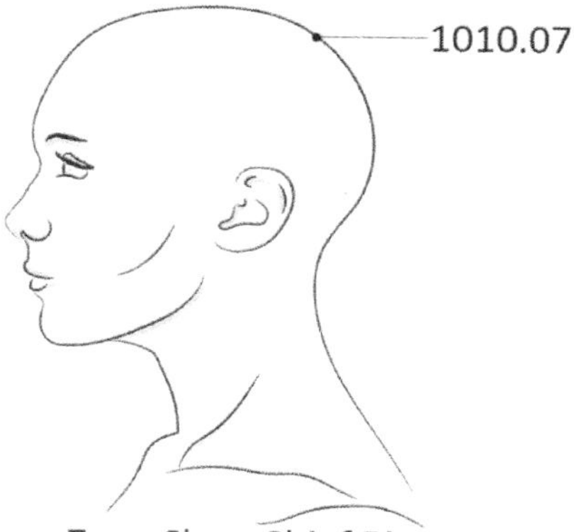

Zong Shu - Chief Pivot

Indications: Vomiting, aphasia, palpitations, neck pain, heart failure.

Reaction area: Dan Tien

Location: .9 cun above the posterior hairline. Superficial insertion, .1 cun deep. Dr. Young suggests bloodletting.

1010.08

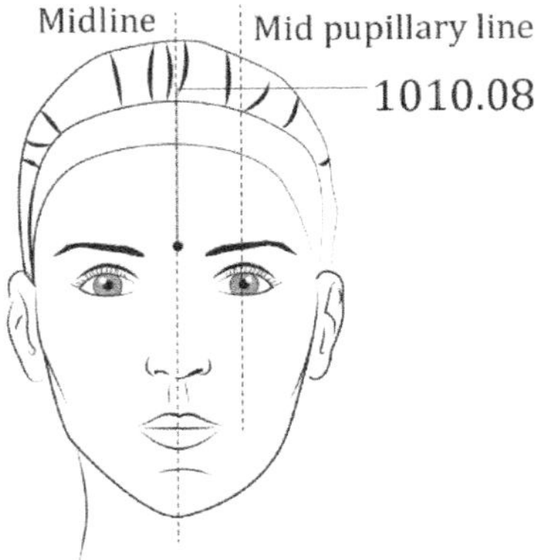

Zhen Jing - Tranquil and Still

Indications: Mental and stress disorders, tremor of limbs, weakness of legs, insomnia, nightmares, restless legs, and limb paralysis.

Reaction area: Brain

Location: One third of a cun above the midpoint between the eyebrows. Insert the needle subcutaneously towards the nose from of 0.1-0.2 cun.

1010.09

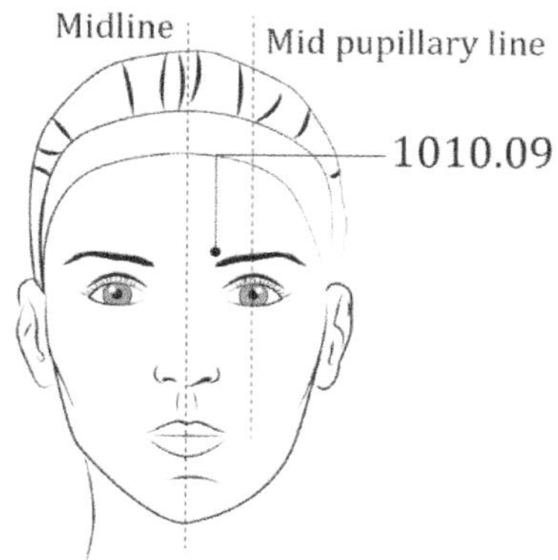

Shang Li - Upper Mile

Indications: Headaches and dizziness.

Location: .2 cun above the medial end of the eyebrow.

1010.10

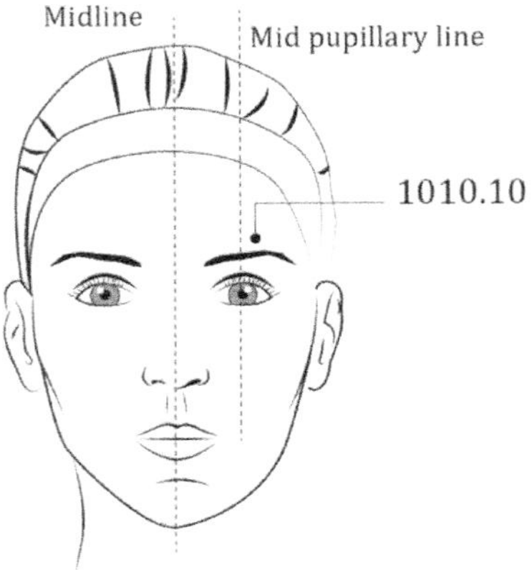

Si Fu Er - Four Bowels Second Point

Indications: Dizziness, headache, and abdominal distension.

Location: .2 cun above the center of the eyebrow.

1010.11

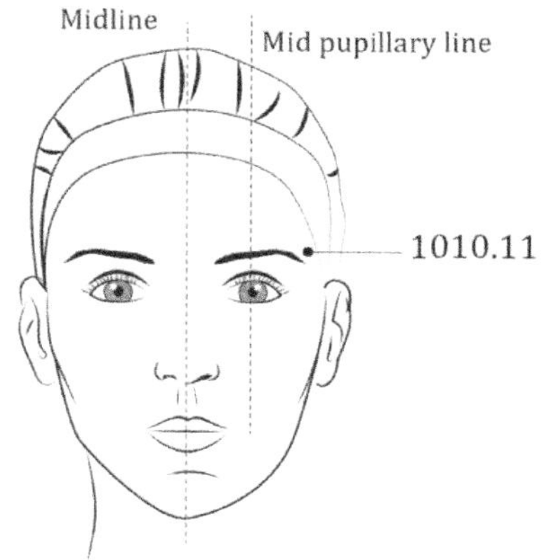

Si Fu Yi - Four Bowels First Point

Indications: Blurred vision, headache, and abdominal distension.

Location: .2 cun above the lateral end of the eyebrow.

1010.12

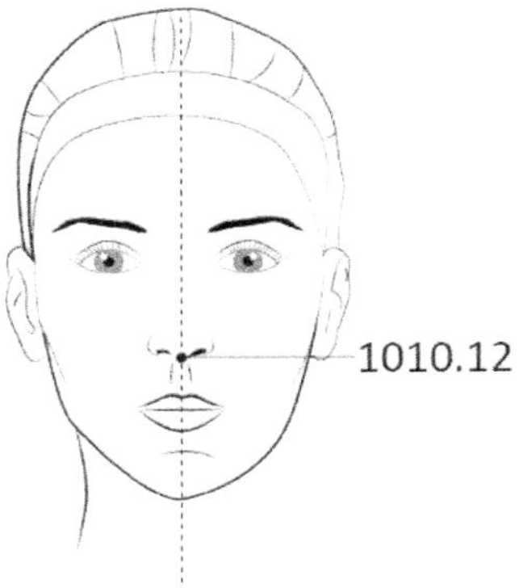

Zheng Ben - Upright Root

Indications: Allergies and psychosis.

Location: Tip of the nose.

1010.13

Ma Jin Shui - Horse Metal Water

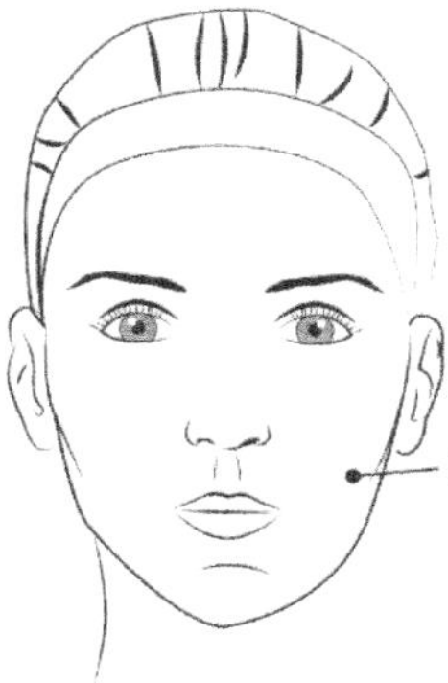

Indications: Nephritis, kidney stones, lower back pain, sciatica, chest pain, regulating free flow of Qi and water metabolism. Promoting the kidney and moving Qi. Regulating the kidney and prostate.

Reaction areas: Kidney, Lung

Locations: Located in the depression beneath the lower border of the zygomatic bone, directly below the outer canthus. Insert perpendicularly at 0.1-0.3 cun deep.

1010.13, 1010.14

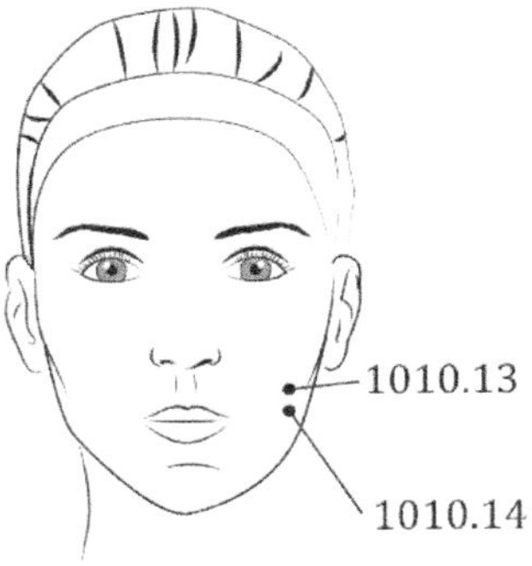

1010.14

Ma Kuai Shui - Horse Fast Water

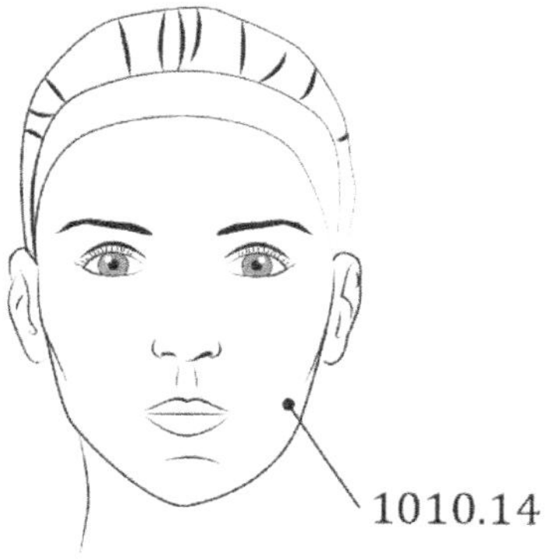

Indications: Bladder stones, cystitis, frequent urination, lumbar pain, and rhinitis.

Reaction areas: Kidney, Bladder

Location: Located .4 cun below, 1010.13.

1010.15

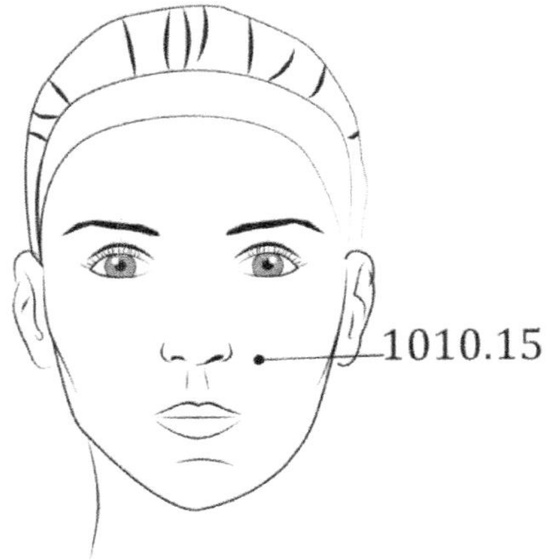

Indications: Abdominal distension and pain, and hernia.

Location: .5 cun below the side of the nostrils. Insertion is .1 to .3 cun.

1010.16

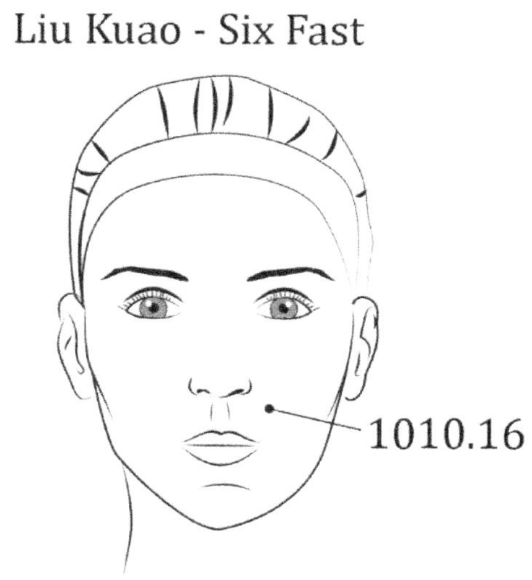

Indications: Ureter stones, and urethritis.

Location: 1.4 cun lateral to the midpoint of the philtrum groove. Insertion is .1 to .3 cun.

1010.17

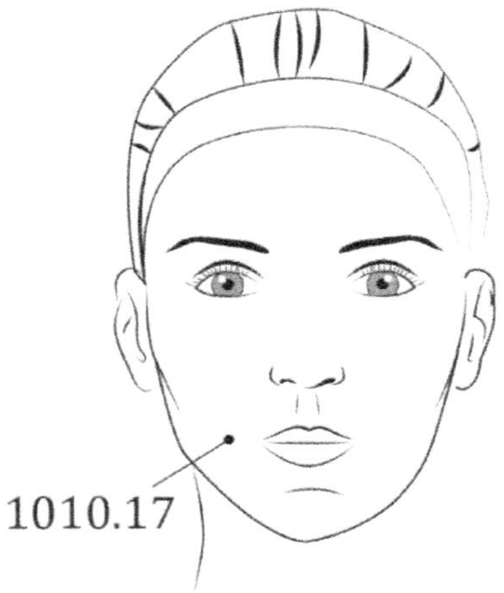

Indications: Facial paralysis, weak lungs, and ureter stone.

Location: .5 cun lateral to the corner of the mouth.

1010.18

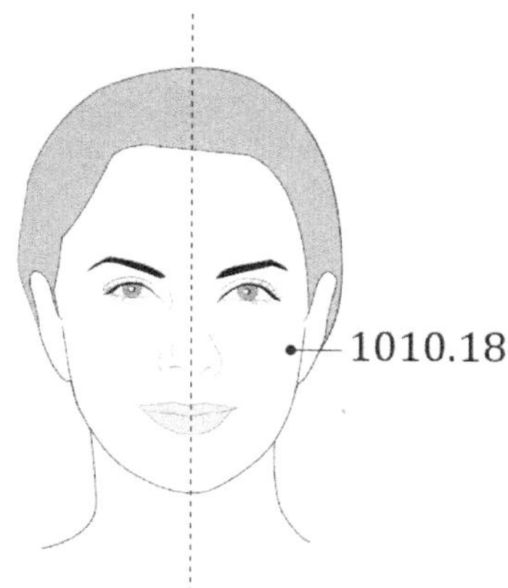

Mu Zhi - Wood Branch

Indications: Liver or gallbladder weakness, gallstones, night crying of babies.

Location: 1 cun lateral to and superior to 1010.13.

1010.19

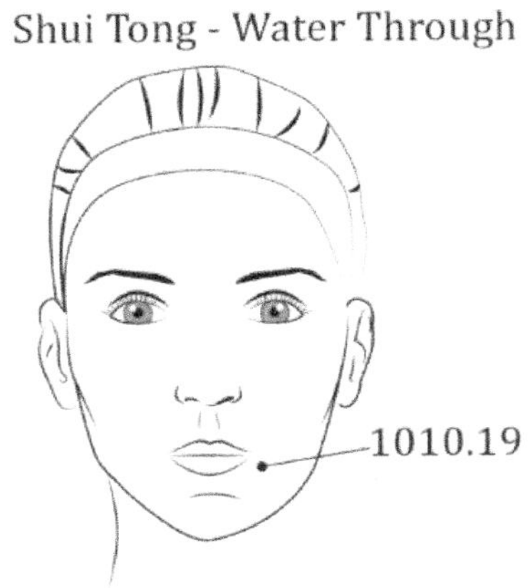

Indications: Lower back pain, acute lumbar sprain, vertigo, dizziness, fatigue, difficulty breathing, and asthma.

Reaction area: Kidney

Location: Half cun below the corner of the mouth. 1010.19 and 1010.20 are often treated with the same needle.

1010.20

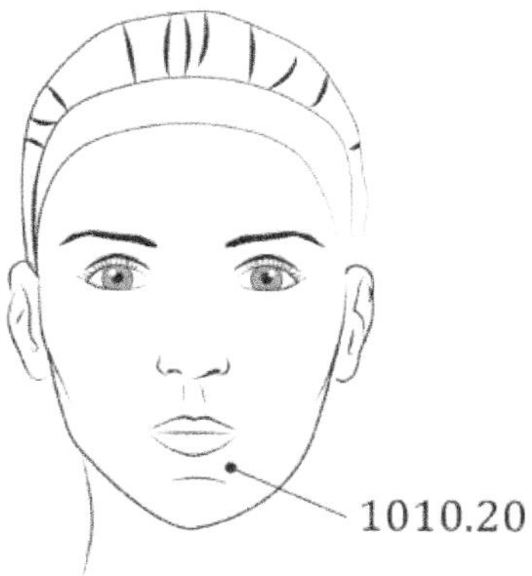

Indications: Lower back pain, acute lumbar sprain, vertigo, dizziness, fatigue, difficulty breathing, and asthma.

Reaction area: Kidney

Location: Located a half cun medial and a 45 degree angle to 1010.19. Some authors thread one needle from 1010.19 to 1010.20. This point is usually combined with 1010.19.

1010.21

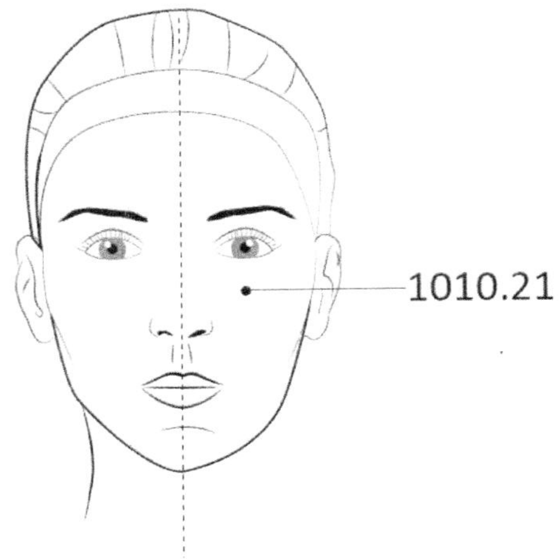

Yu Hou - Jade Fire

Indications: Sciatica, knee pain, shoulder pain, cheek pain, upper jawbone pain.

Reaction areas: Heart, Liver

Location: Directly below the pupil, in the depression below the zygomatic bone.

1010.22

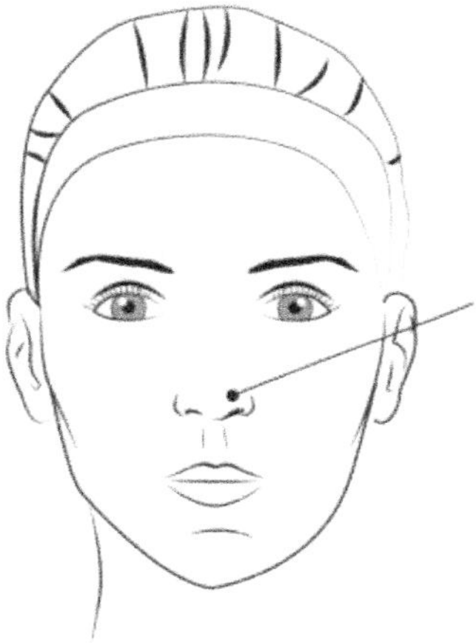

Indications: Migraines, vertigo, facial paralysis, supraorbital pain, a tongue that is painful, stiff, or tight, sore throat.

Reaction areas: Lung, Kidney, Spleen

Location: At the superior border of the nostril, in the depression.

1010.23, 1010.24

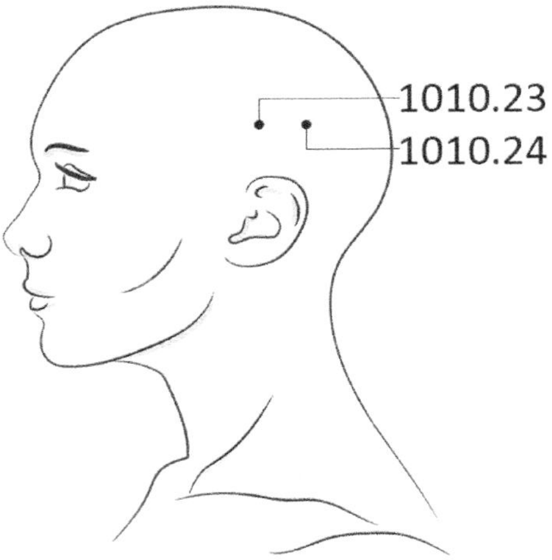

1010.23, Zhou Huo, Prefecture Fire

Indications: Lower back pain, palpitations, fatigue, arthritis.

Location: 1.5 cun above the ear apex

1010.24, Zhou Jin, Prefecture Metal

Indications: Sciatica, lower back pain, arthritis.

Location: 1 cun posterior to 1010.23

1010.25

Zhou Shui - Prefecture Water

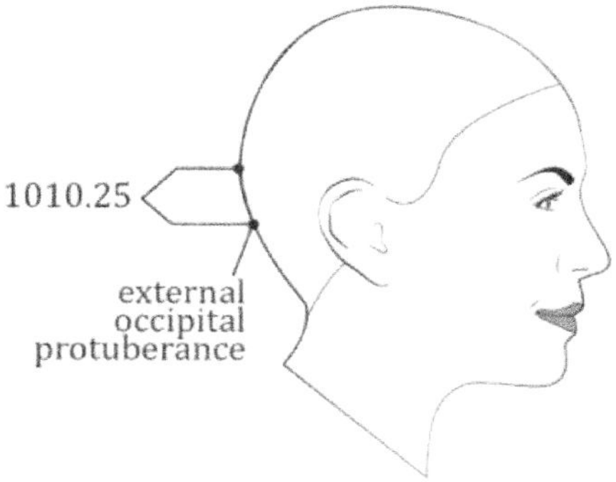

Indications: Spine pain, leg paralysis. These two indications are the most commonly cited. However, Brad Whisnant has expounded on this point in his book*, Top Tung Acupuncture Points*. He also wrote a book called *Treat Back Pain Distally*, which is an excellent guide to using the Balance Method, and Tung points to treat back pain, sciatica, and hip pain.

Brad Whisnant uses these points to treat sciatica, spinal stenosis, compression, bone spurs, foramen narrowing, disc degeneration and compression, radiculopathy, piriformis syndrome, ischial tuberosity pain, sacral pain, and PSIS pain. Brad says that these points are extremely effective to treat lower back pain on the sacrum.

1010.25

This point is one of the few points that treats foramen narrowing. The external occipital protuberance images the sacrum. I will refer you to the book *Top Tung Acupuncture Points*, for an in depth analysis of this point, as well as treatment notes.

Reaction area: Kidney

Location: The first point of this two point unit is just above the EOP, or external occipital protuberance. The second point is .8 cun superior to that. Thread a single needle from the second point to the first point. Insertion is .8 cun.

An insertion trick from Brad Whisnant is to press on the skin at the tip of the needle as you insert it. The needle will glide in easily as you use this insertion technique. If it gets stuck, pull it out a bit and re-insert.

Unnumbered Tung Points

Ci Bai

Sequence White

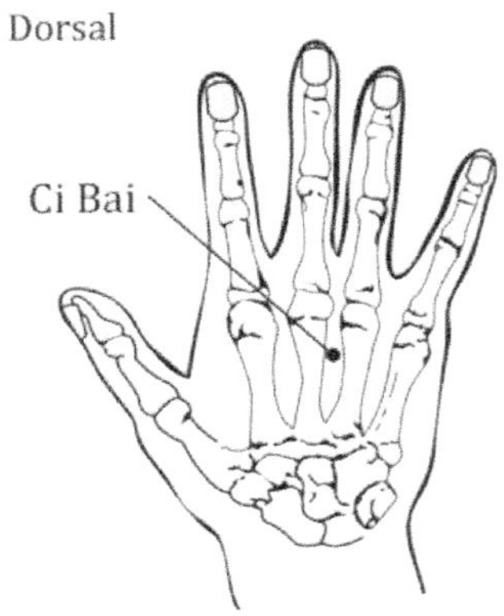

Indications: Headaches, neck pain, leg pain, and lower back pain.

Locations: .5 cun posterior to junction of third and fourth metacarpal bones, at the same level as SJ 3. Insertion is .5 cun.

Fan Hou Jue

Cutting Opposite and Behind

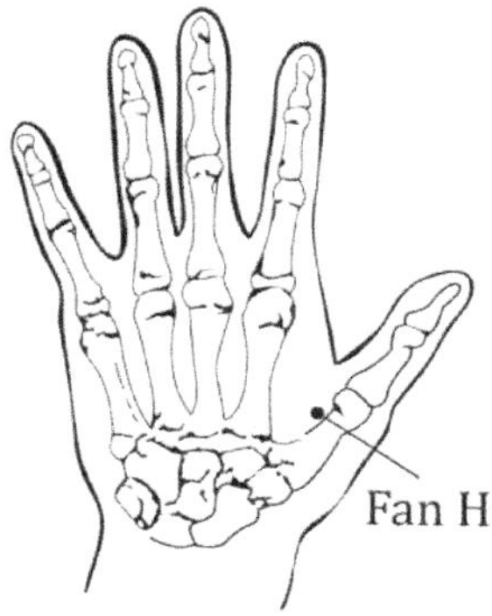

Indications: Shoulder pain, stiff upper back and shoulders. It is famous for shoulder pain. Brad Whisnant refers to this as his first choice to treat shoulder pain. He combines Fan Hou Jue, Ling Gu, and Da Bai.

Reaction area: Lung

Location: This point is located on the hand dorsum, one cun distal to Ling Gu. Insert the needle close to the thumb metacarpal bone.

Fu Ge San

Bowel Grid Three

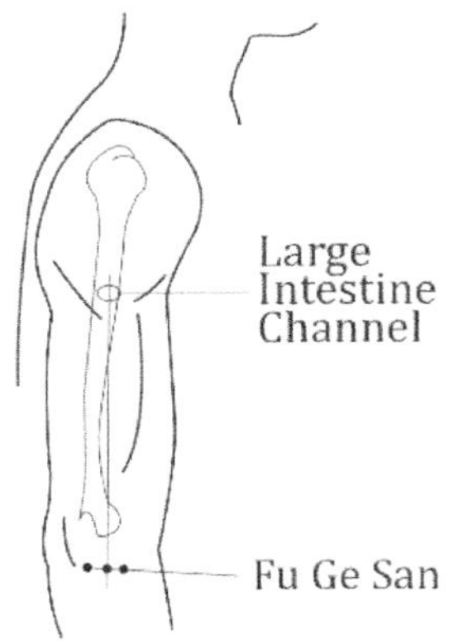

Indications: Severe common cold.

Reaction Areas: Heart, Lung

Location: A three point unit. First point is .8 cun distal to LI 11. The other two points are .8 cun to the left and right of the first point.

Gu Ci Yi Er San

Bone Spur Points

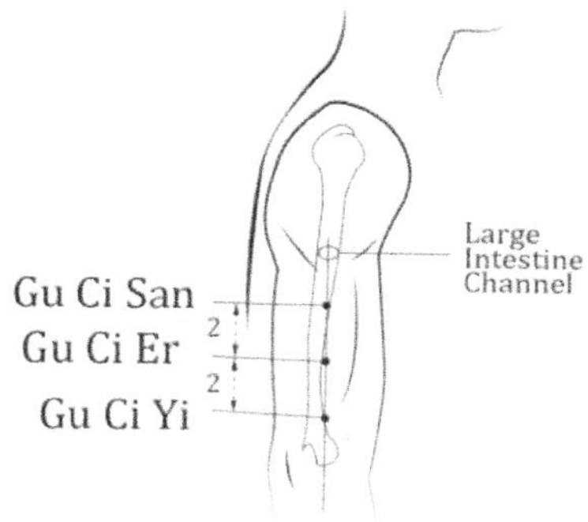

Bone Spur Points

Indications: Bone spurs, pain and traumatic injury of the vertebrae.

Reaction Areas: Liver, Kidney. (Most sources list Gu Ci San as only the Liver)

Location: Gu Ci Yi is the first point, Gu Ci Er is 2 cun proximal from that, and Gu Ci San is 2 cun from Gu Ci Er.

Gu Guan, Mu Guan

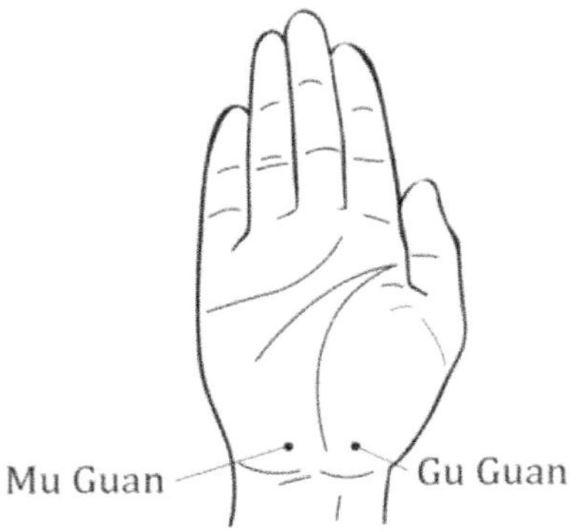

Gu Guan, Bone Gate
Mu Guan, Wood Gate

Indications: Heel pain, joint swelling, arthritis, and bone swelling.

Reaction areas: Both points are Kidney and Lung

Location: Mu Guan is located at the base of the palm, .5 cun distal to the pisiform bone. Gu Guan is located at the base of the palm, in the depression .5 cun distal to the scaphoid bone. For best results, tap the bone with your needle.

Pian Jian

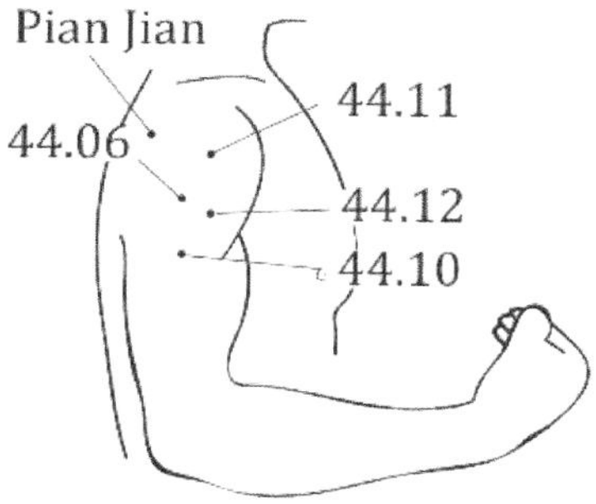

Indications: Sciatica

Location: One source says it is 1 cun posterior to LI 15, another source says it is located at TCM LI 15.

San Cha Er

Three Jam, Two

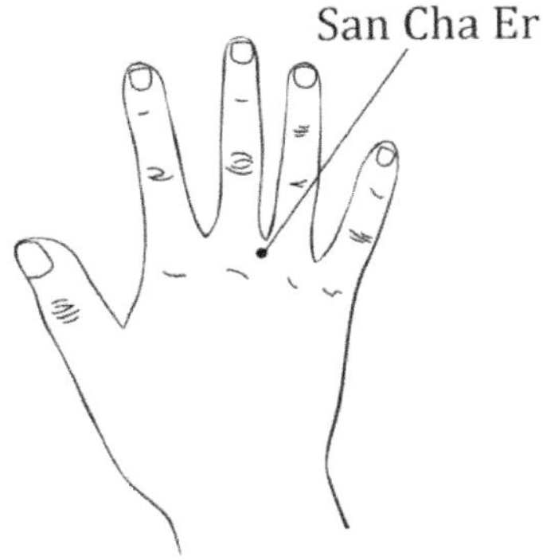

Indications: Neck pain, knee pain, back pain, opens the five sense organs, ear pain, headaches, benefits the heart.

Location: at the junction of the third and fourth fingers. Insertion is 1 to 1.5 cun.

San Cha San

Three Openings, Three

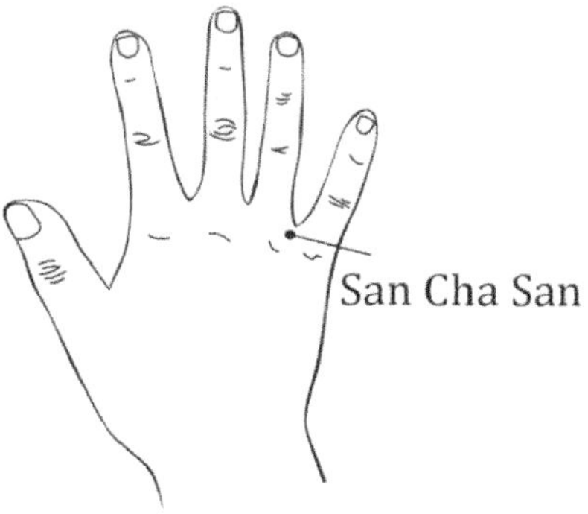

Indications: Knee pain, acute lumbar sprain, and diseases of the five sense organs. It also strengthens the heart. Common cold, headaches, shoulder pain, tinnitus, palpitations, hives, leg pain, fatigue, spleen Qi issues. It opens the five orifices of the face, treats heavy eyes, sweating, weak muscles, and thigh pain.

Reaction areas: Spleen, Kidney

Location: Between the fourth and fifth fingers. Insertion is 1 to 1.5 cun.

San Cha Yi

Three Jam, One

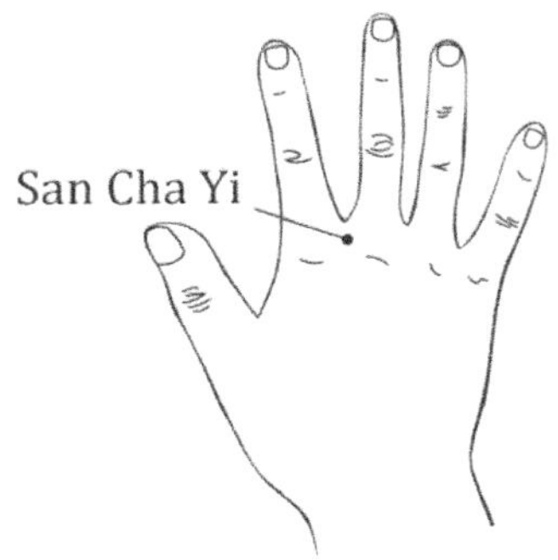

Indications: Hip and lower back pain, shoulder pain, neck pain, stomach pain, irregular menses, regulates and strengthens the lungs. Often combined with San Cha Er and San for back and hip pain.

Location: At the junction of the second and third fingers.

Tou Points

Ding Tou, Hou Tou, Pian Tou, Qian Tou

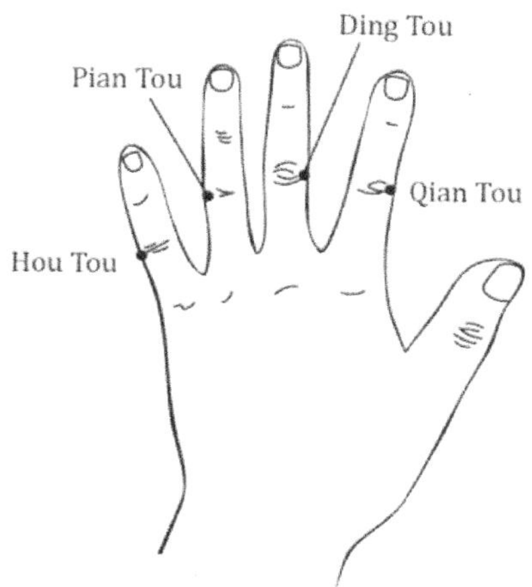

Indications: Headaches.

Locations:
Qian Tou and Ding Tou are needled in the direction of the little finger.
Pian Tou and Hou Tou are needled in the direction of the thumb.

All needles are perpendicular and the points are located where the pink and white skin meet. Touch the bone on insertion. Since we are treating the skull, the needle should touch the bone to be effective.

Tou Points

Ding Tou, Hou Tou, Pian Tou, Qian Tou

If you want to use one Tou point at a time, these are the locations they treat:

Qian Tou – Frontal headaches
Ding Tou – Vertex headaches
Pian Tou – Parietal headaches
Hou Tou – Occipital headaches

These points are from the book *Advanced Tung Style Acupuncture: Anesthesiology/Pain Management* by Dr. James H. Maher. This book contains Tung points that are not available elsewhere, as well as treatment protocols. I highly recommend it. Dr. Maher translated numerous Tung texts from Chinese into English. He has written eight books on Tung acupuncture.

Xiao Jie

Small Joint

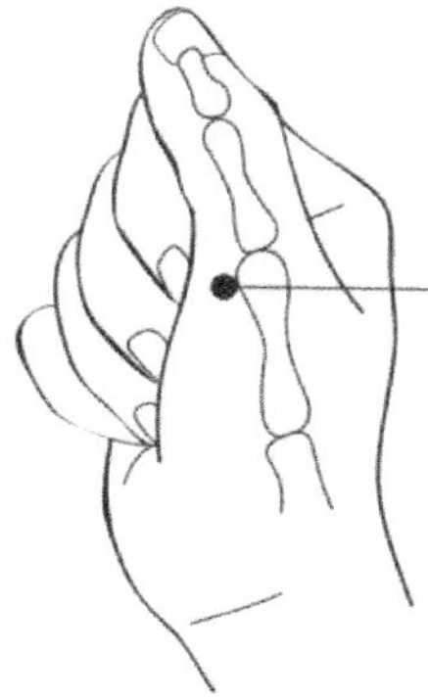

Indications: Ankle pain, especially on the medial side of the ankle. Dr. Young cites it as being effective for neck pain, shoulder pain, back pain, sciatica, chest pain, stomachache, chronic diarrhea, and pain of the elbow and wrist.

Reaction areas: Lung, Heart

Location: Located on the side of the first metacarpal bone, at the junction of the red and white skin. Insertion is 1 to 1.5 cun.

Ye Mang

Night Blindness

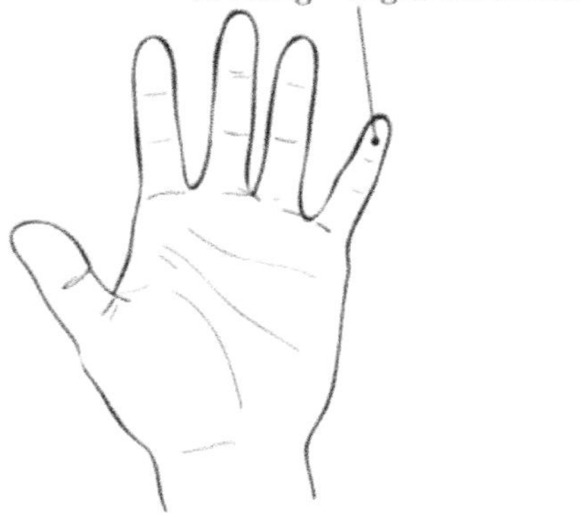

Indication: Night blindness.

Location: On the little finger, at the midpoint of the distal finger crease. Insertion is .2 cun.

Zhi Han

Stop Sweating

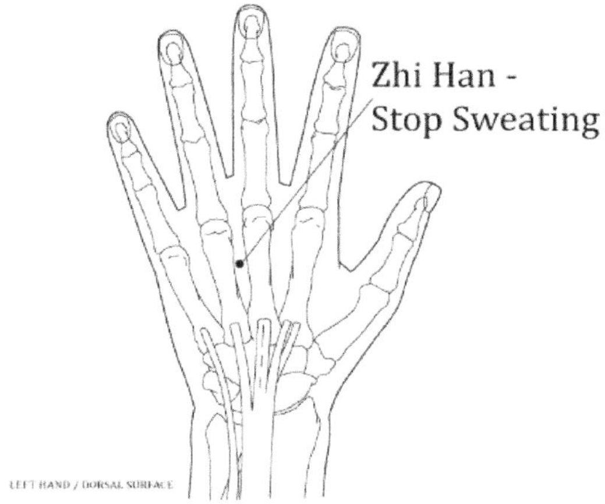

Indications: Stop sweating

Reaction areas: Liver, Spleen

Location: Dorsum of the hand, between the third and fourth metacarpal bones.

This point was found in the book *Practical Atlas of Tung's Acupuncture*, by Henry McCann, and Hans-Georg Ross. They refer to it as a special point from Dr. Hu Bing Quan. This is an example of how many points there are in the Tung system. You cannot get all the points by buying one book.

References

Advanced Tung Style Acupuncture: The Dao Ma Needling Technique of Master Tung Ching Chang
Advanced Tung Style Acupuncture: Anesthesiology/Pain Management, 2005
Dr. James H. Maher

Lectures on Tung's Acupuncture – Points Study, 2008
Tung's Acupuncture, 2005
Lectures on Tung's Acupuncture Therapeutic System, 2008
Dr. Wei Chieh Young

Top Tung Acupuncture Points, 2015
Treat Back Pain Distally, 2015
Brad Whisnant

Practical Atlas of Tung's Acupuncture – 2014
Henry McCann and Hans-Georg Ross

Introduction to Tung's Acupuncture – 2014
Dr. Chuan-Min Wang DC L.Ac. (Author), Steven Vasilakis LAc (Editor)

Master Tung's Acupuncture: An Ancient Alternative Style in Modern Clinical Practice, Oct 1992
Miriam Lee

INDEX

abdominal pain, 28, 63, 65, 93, 149
abscesses, 46, 131
allergies, 62, 72
amenorrhea, 52
anger, 37
angina, 89
ankle pain, 197
aphasia, 152, 153, 154, 159, 165
aphonia, 155
appendicitis, 99
arm pain, 69, 78, 87, 88, 91, 120, 122, 125
arm paralysis, 30
armpit odor, 83
arteriosclerosis, 76, 79
arthritis, 36, 122, 182, 190
asthma, 48, 49, 51, 62, 69, 71, 78, 114, 115, 116, 143, 161, 162, 178, 179
astigmatism, 53, 132
bladder stones, 173
bleeding, stops, 102, 103
blurred vision, 54, 55, 56, 62, 65, 105, 106, 139, 141, 142, 163
bone enlargement, 42
bone spurs, 118, 148, 183, 189
bone tuberculosis, 164
brain tumor, 94, 112, 162
breast pain, 143
breath, shortness, 161, 162
breech presentation, 98
bronchitis, 23
calf pain, 31, 80, 83
carditis, 116
carpal tunnel syndrome, 61, 88
cataracts, 108, 109, 132
cerebellum swelling, 94
cerebral ischemia, 133
cerebral palsy, 159
cheek pain, 180
chest, 25, 61, 130
chest pain, 48, 49, 143, 171, 197
chest stuffiness, 23
cholera, 68, 158
chorea, 139
cirrhosis, 40, 139
clavicle pain, 130
coccyx pain, 68
common cold, 37, 62, 69, 78, 137, 158, 188

gallbladder, 33, 100, 101, 141, 177
gallstones, 100, 141, 142, 177
gastritis, 58
genital, 37, 123
glaucoma, 32, 132
gout, 47
groin pain, 68
hand cramps, 61
hand pain, 125
hands, 37, 98, 144, 152, 153, 154
headaches, 32, 54, 102, 103, 112, 148, 164, 192, 193, 196
hearing, 90, 145
heart, 23, 29, 31, 49, 53, 54, 57, 60, 68, 69, 71, 73, 74, 75, 76, 96, 97, 98, 104, 105, 106, 112, 114, 115, 116, 119, 122, 133, 140, 156, 180, 188, 197
heart attacks emergency point, 98
heart deficiency, 35
heart disease, 39, 79
heart failure, 156, 165
heart inflammation, 68
heart pain, 50, 115, 116
heel pain, 127, 190
hematuria, 123, 124, 126
hemiplegia, 30, 52, 76, 86, 143, 148, 152, 153, 154, 159, 161, 162
hemorrhoid pain, 59
hepatitis, 40, 65, 67, 139
hepatocirrhosis, 157
hepatomegaly, 157
hernia, 23, 24, 37, 95, 174
hoarse voice, 155
hydrocephalus, 110
hypertension, 54, 73, 74, 75, 84, 85, 86, 87, 104, 105, 120, 122
impotence, 123, 124, 126
indigestion, 100, 101, 139, 147
infertility, 44, 96
instep pain, 120
intercostal neuralgia, 120
intestinal pain, 52, 135, 136
intraocular eye pressure, 32
irritability, 37
ischial tuberosity pain, 183
jaundice, 43, 78
joints, achy, 47
kidney pain, 32
kidney stones, 88, 171
knee osteoarthritis, 119
knee pain, 23, 25, 29, 33, 36, 49, 68, 76, 148, 180, 192, 193
laryngitis, 72, 77, 128, 131
lateral malleolus pain, 53
leg muscle pain, 88
leg pain, 62, 63, 78, 80, 87, 150, 186, 193

leucorrhea, 26, 80, 82
limb weakness, 152, 153, 154
lip pain, 121
liver disease, 98, 100, 112
Liver Fire, 37
liver pain, 54, 139
liver, swollen, 40
lumbar pain, 31, 173
macular degeneration, 32
mastitis, 112
menstruation, irregular, 26, 44, 52, 96, 123, 124, 126
migraine, 52, 102, 103, 112, 120, 148, 158, 181
miscarriage, 26
mouth ulcerations, 121
mumps, 131
muscle atrophy, 34
muscle spasms, 71
nausea, 77, 133
neck pain, 31, 49, 75, 103, 106, 110, 148, 165, 186, 194, 197
neck stiff, 110
neck, stiff, 105
needle shock, 57
nephritis, 55, 56, 73, 88, 108, 109, 122, 123, 124, 126, 138, 171
neuropathy, 132
night blindness, 198
night crying, 33, 177
nightmares, 33, 166
nocturnal emission, 123, 124, 126
nose, congested, 37
nosebleeds, 32, 56, 76, 94
osteoarthritis, 42
otitis, 143
palpitations, 23, 25, 39, 49, 54, 60, 68, 71, 76, 97, 104, 105, 114, 119, 133, 152, 153, 154, 165, 182, 193
parathyroiditis, 155
pelvic pain, 44
pericarditis, 133
photophobia, 105
placenta, retention of, 89, 97
pleura, 27
pleurisy, 27, 130, 143
plum pit Qi, 128
pneumonia, 47, 48, 49, 143
polio, 76, 80, 82, 83, 86, 87, 100, 101
polycythemia, 156
pre-eclampsia, 108, 109
pregnancy, 44, 51, 52, 133
prostate, 123, 171
proteinuria, 122, 123, 124, 126
PSIS pain, 183
psoriasis, 143
psychosis, 170
rectal prolapse, 59, 99
respiratory problems, 37
retinopathy, 132

rheumatic fever, 133
rheumatic heart disease, 36, 133
rhinitis, 27, 69, 143, 173
rib pain, 112, 130, 143
sacral pain, 68, 183
sacral vertebral pain, 31
scanty menstruation, 44
scapula pain, 29
sciatica, 50, 51, 52, 53, 55, 56, 62, 63, 68, 77, 86, 87, 92, 93, 110, 120, 143, 158, 161, 162, 171, 180, 182, 183, 191, 197
scrofula, 47
seminal emission, 123, 124, 126
shoulder pain, 29, 69, 76, 128, 129, 180, 187, 193, 194, 197
sinus, 37
sinusitis, 62, 127
skin allergies, 147
skin diseases, 76
small intestine inflammation, 23, 99
sore throat, 47, 181
spinal pain, 56, 92, 110, 164
spine pain, 108, 109
spleen, 38, 78, 193
splenomegaly, 101, 112
sternum pain, 130
stomach disease, 58, 98
stomach hemorrhage, 135, 136
stomach pain, 24, 115, 116, 118, 194
strangury, 123, 124, 126, 157
stress, 37, 97, 166
stroke, 152, 153, 154, 159, 164
supraorbital bone, 32
sweating, stop, 199
teeth grinding, 117
tennis elbow, 120
thigh pain, 68, 148, 150, 193
thirst, 35
throat abscess, 128, 129
thyroiditis, 128, 155
tinnitus, 27, 52, 54, 56, 90, 143, 145, 148, 193
TMJ, 97
toe pain, 47
tongue, 181
tonsillitis, 112, 128, 131, 155, 158
toothache, 24, 54, 90, 114, 120, 127
trachoma, 90
transient ischemic attacks, 152, 153, 154
trigeminal neuralgia, 56, 94, 123, 126, 127
tuberculosis, 143
tumors, 98, 107, 112, 124, 131, 135, 136
ulcer, 58

Other books:

Acupuncture Points Handbook is a compilation of numerous acupuncture texts. It has over 400 acupuncture points. It was written with patient needs in mind. Each point is explained in layman's terms and TCM terms. Acupressure and basic info on how acupuncture works is at the front of the book. *Acupuncture Points Quick Guide* is an excerpt of that, which includes only the most commonly used points.

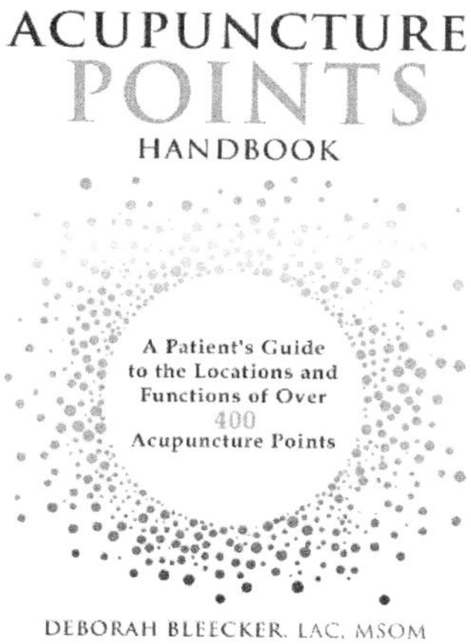

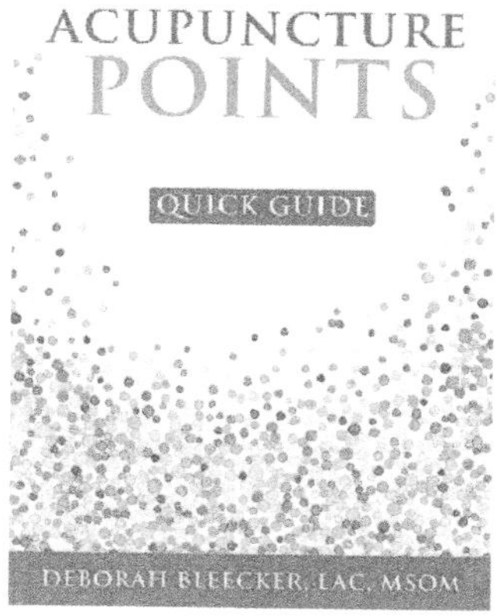

Contact

I would love to hear from you. You can reach me at deborahbleecker@gmail.com.

Printed in Great Britain
by Amazon

58256676R00119